THE NEW

HEART DISEASE

A practical guide to all aspects of heart disease and
its prevention, with invaluable advice for all those
who want to enjoy good health and long life.

By the same author

THE NEW SELF HELP SERIES

HEART DISEASE

A PRACTICAL GUIDE TO ALL
ASPECTS OF HEART DISEASE
AND ITS PREVENTION

LEONARD MERVYN
B.Sc. Ph.D. C.Chem. F.R.S.C.

Thorsons
An Imprint of HarperCollinsPublishers

Thorsons
An Imprint of HarperCollins*Publishers*
77–85 Fulham Palace Road,
Hammersmith, London W6 8JB
1160 Battery Street, San Francisco,
California 94111–1213

First published in *The Science of Life* series
This edition published by Thorsons 1990
3   5   7   9   10   8   6   4   2

© Leonard Mervyn 1930

Leonard Mervyn asserts the moral right to
be identified as the author of this work

A catalogue record for this book
is available from the British Library

ISBN 0 7225 2256 8

Printed in Great Britain by
HarperCollinsManufacturing Glasgow

Contents

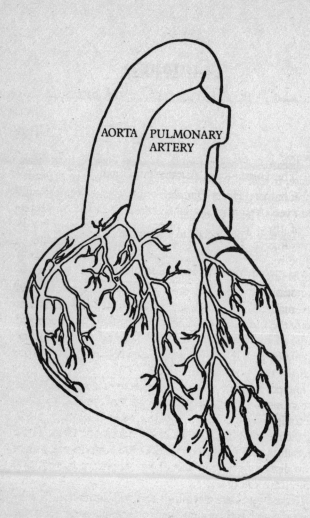

An illustration of the distribution of the coronary arteries. They carry blood to all portions of the heart muscle.

1

The Heart
— An Astounding Organ

No disease is more common or more deadly than heart disease, in one of its varied forms. Every year in Australia almost half of the deaths are due to diseases of the heart and blood vessels (cardiovascular disease). Over 50,000 people die of these ailments in Australia every year! That is approximately 1,000 every week, or 4,000 per month.

The road safety authorities are shocked because 3,000 people are killed on the road every year, but more cardiovascular cases die every month, and most of it is preventable. If this death rate is maintained, it means that nearly every second person alive in Australia today is doomed to die of heart disease or a 'stroke'. In other words some 5,000,000 people now living in Australia are doomed to die of heart trouble or hypertension.

The position is much the same in Britain and the USA. According to a round table conference of the leading heart specialists of America held in December 1979, there are in the vicinity of 25,000,000 heart sufferers in the USA. These specialists have estimated that 800,000 Americans contract heart disease every year and each year approximately 650,000 Americans die of it.

These figures are alarming. You will naturally ask, why heart disease? Is there something organically weak about the human heart in comparison with the other organs? No. On the contrary, the heart is a notoriously strong organ. In fact, it is the most powerful muscular organ in the body. On and on it must beat—72 times a minute, 4,320 beats per hour, 37,843,200 per year! And the heart performs that amazing task for 50, 60, 70, 80 or 100 years or more.

Anatomy of the heart

The heart is a muscular pump about the size of a fist and it weighs about 10 oz. To sustain life it has to beat about forty million times a year. It supplies blood to every organ and tissue in the body, including itself. The heart obtains no nourishment from the blood as it passes through its pumping chambers but the heart muscle receives its blood and hence oxygen supply through two small arteries about an eighth of an inch in diameter. These arteries, called coronary arteries, arise from the main exit channel of the heart, called the aorta. Backflow of blood from these arteries to the heart is prevented by an aortic valve.

The three important parts of the heart's structure are:
(1) The muscle that contracts and pumps the blood;
(2) The valves through which the blood enters and leaves the heart;
(3) The blood vessels (coronary arteries) that carry oxygen and nourishment to the heart muscle.

The heart consists of four chambers: the left and right ventricle, and the left and right auricle, also called left and right atrium—atrium means the first chamber. The walls of all four chambers consist of muscle.

Circulation of the blood

The veins carry blood that has had part of its oxygen removed by the various tissues and organs of the body and this venous blood is collected and fed into the right auricle. The auricle contracts and pushes the venous blood into the right ventricle which also contracts, channelling the blood into the vascular (blood vessel) system of the lungs. Here it is renewed with oxygen (by respiration) and carbon dioxide is removed so that blood leaving the lungs is brighter and redder than that entering them. From the lungs, the oxygenated blood is pushed into the left auricle which contracts forcing it into the left ventricle. From here, the blood is distributed to all the tissues and organs, (including the heart) via the arteries so bringing a fresh supply of oxygen for metabolic needs. The fresh oxygen in the arteries exchanges with carbon dioxide, which is a waste product of metabolism, and this blood is directed via the veins back into the right side of the heart. The whole cycle then continues in the same way.

The quantity of blood pumped by the heart varies from hour to hour. Even while we rest, the heart expels from 2½ to 4 oz of blood from each ventricle with every contraction. If you multiply this figure by 70, which is the average number of contractions per minute, you find that the output of blood pumped by the heart is about 4 qt for both ventricles per minute—which is 60 gal per hour, or 1,440 gal per day! To carry this mathematical exercise further and multiply the above figure by the days in the year, we get a figure bordering on the astronomical. And this prodigious task is performed by a sturdy muscular mechanism slightly larger than a closed fist! In terms of weight, there is certainly something astonishing about a small fist-sized organ that pumps over 11 tons of blood through an adult human body every twenty-four hours. ELEVEN TONS!

This fact is probably the most staggering of all the amazing facts of the human body. Those who conclude from the foregoing facts and figures that the rising incidence of heart failure is due to this organ breaking down under constant strain are completely wrong. The average physical worker whose heart each working day works twice, three times and four times as hard as that of the sedentary worker or housewife, does not add seriously to the ranks of heart cases. The average man doing hard physical work has the best record, from the point of view of heart disease, of all the professions and avocations.

It is vitally important that you understand why and how the circulatory mechanism in general and the heart in particular becomes silted up.

Spend a few minutes studying the diagram of the heart on page 6.

You will notice a network of arteries on the outside of the heart. This is an anterior view. There is also a network of arteries, veins and tiny blood capillaries throughout the heart muscle. The arteries which you can see in the diagram (and a network of arteries which you cannot see) are called coronary arteries. These coronary arteries feed the heart muscle. They carry blood to all portions of the heart muscle.

Now turn to the illustration on page 16 and note how these arteries are silted up, making it difficult for the blood to flow through. What are these deposits in the coronary arteries and how do they come about? These deposits are partly uric acid deposits—acid urates, xanthine, hypoxanthine, creatine, and others. They are the end products of wrong feeding, of excess protein (meat and eggs chiefly), white bread, condiments, pickled vegetables, corned meat, toasted and processed breakfast cereals, strong tea and coffee, sugar, jam processed desserts, sausage meats, pastry and confectionery, sweetened foods, etc. In addition of course the deposits are often overlaid with fats and cholesterol and we shall see later how this deposition may be avoided.

The coronary arteries
Let us now look in more detail at the coronary arteries, those vital blood vessels that convey the blood to the heart muscle itself.

The initial course of the coronary arteries lies in the groove between the receiving (auricle) and pumping (ventricle) chambers of the heart. From this groove branches descend over the surface of the heart (see diagram on page 6) and smaller ones arise from these and penetrate the heart muscle. When the heart was studied by the first anatomists, they saw that this pattern of blood vessels resembled a crown (coron) so they were termed coronary arteries. Once the blood from these arteries has supplied oxygen to the heart muscle and picked up carbon dioxide and other waste nutrients, it is drained into the heart itself. Then via the organ it is sent back to the lungs for a further supply of oxygen like any venous blood.

Coronary artery disease

In the new-born child, the inner lining of the coronary arteries is smooth, glistening and pearly white. The arteries themselves have a supple wall of muscle and elastic tissue which enables them to respond to and indeed contribute to maintenance of the blood-pressure. If our coronary arteries retained this suppleness throughout life, coronary artery disease would never happen but unfortunately as we grow older this healthy condition gradually deteriorates. The end-result is the most prevalent form of heart disease, accounting for more illness and deaths than any other heart condition. Coronary heart disease is now so common that there can hardly be a family without at least one member being affected by it.

How is the coronary artery damaged?

In those who are affected, the artery lining becomes gradually discoloured, thickened and roughened by an increase in the number of cells in the wall. At the same time there is deposition of fatty material and various other components of the blood (see above) which are deposited in or on it. Consequently, the inside diameter of the vessel is reduced in places and the artery loses its elasticity. The condition is known as atherosclerosis, a word derived from the Greek athero, meaning gruel, and sclerosis, meaning hardening. This apt combination describes neatly the major changes in the arterial wall. A more popular term for the condition is hardening of the arteries.

Post mortems show these deposits to be almost as hard as slate. The slow silting-up of the whole circulatory mechanism may take 40, 50, 60 or 70 years before it brings about the inevitable degeneracy burden placed on the heart when the blood vessels of the body are silted up. It is still obliged to pump the entire blood supply through these half-closed pipes. But to do so it must pump much harder. Is it any wonder that the heart muscle so frequently breaks down under the strain?

These changes develop in most people as they get older but in some the process is more rapid and severe. It is only when the arterial tube is greatly narrowed to the extent of about three-quarters of its cross-sectional area that serious obstruction to blood flow results. When this happens, the area of muscle supplied by the artery is deprived of its normal quota of blood and hence oxygen and so it suffers. It can be so bad that death of that area of muscle results and the result is known as an infarct.

These changes are not confined to the coronary arteries—the blood vessels in other parts of the body may also be affected. When the arteries supplying blood to the calves of the legs become hardened and silted up, the condition is called Intermittent Claudication, characterized by pain in the calves or thighs on walking. Sometimes the arteries in the brain may be so afflicted that the result can be a stroke where the brain is damaged by deprivation of its blood supply or by a vessel that bursts, causing haemorrhage. In this book however, our main concern is with the arteries supplying the heart.

Methods of detecting heart disease

The electrocardiogram (ECG for short) represents the heart specialist's indispensable tool for determining irregularities in heart function. Small metal plates, known as electrodes, are placed on the limbs and chest and connected to the electrocardiograph machine with wires. When the heart beats, it does so in response to an electrical stimulus produced in the heart itself, and the small electrical current generated is picked up by the electrodes and fed into the machine. This in turn amplifies the tiny current and transfers its variations and strength on to a moving band of paper. The result is the electro-cardiogram, sometimes known as electric heart writing. From the shape of the pattern that emerges, the heart specialist can deduce quite a lot about the heart's functioning.

The electrical impulse originates within specialized pacemaker cells at the junction of the principal vein that drains the upper portion of the body (superior vena cava) and the right auricle. It is known as the sinoatrial (S-A) node and the cells represent the primary electrical generator (pacemaker) for the normal human heart. The impulse from the S-A node then travels over the auricles to another node at the junction of the auricles and ventricles (A-V node). Here it is propagated through a specialized group of conducting fibres called the His bundle. The His bundle itself splits into three major conducting groups of fibres called the right bundle which carries the impulse over the right ventricle and the main left bundle which supplies the impulse to the left side of the heart. This in turn divides into the left posterior division which cascades down the area between the right and left ventricles and the left anterior division which runs to the left ventricle—the main pumping chamber of the heart. In this way the original impulse is spread over the whole of the surface of the heart and it is the electricity induced that causes the heart to beat.

The normal electrocardiogram looks like this with the various waves designated P, QRS and T.

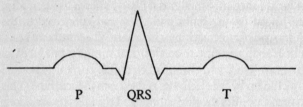

    P   QRS   T

The first or P wave is caused by the passage of the impulse from the S-A node and it stimulates auricular contraction. The QRS and T waves are the result of passage of the impulse from the A-V node and all are related to contraction of the ventricles. The electrocardiogram hence gives important information concerning the spread of excitation to the different chambers of the heart and is of value in the diagnosis of cases of abnormal heart rhythm and any damage to the heart muscle. It can also indicate any enlargement of the heart chambers.

Electrocardiograms do, however, have their limitations. A normal ECG is no guarantee that the individual is free from coronary disease. It is possible for sufferers from angina to have normal ECGs at rest though many will show abnormalities during or after exercise. Even patients with extensive coronary disease and blocked arteries may have normal tracings because these give information only about the spread of electrical activity over the heart. Whilst useful in diagnosing and monitoring the progress of certain heart diseases, the ECG is a fairly crude diagnoser of coronary disease.

Coronary angiography is of more use in this respect. For this investigation, a contrast material (something that will show up on X-rays) is passed via a catheter into the artery of an arm or a leg or even into the heart chambers themselves which are then X-rayed. Using this technique it is possible to observe in detail the state of the heart chambers or blood vessels. Any site of narrowing or obstruction will show up when in contact with the contrast material and this can be pinpointed accurately. Remedial measures can then be undertaken.

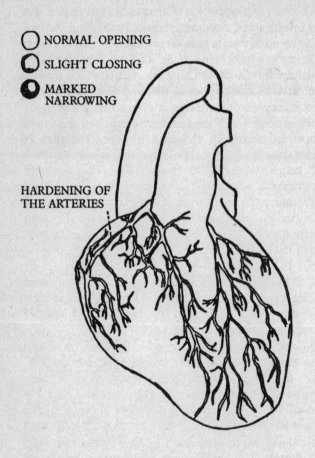

NORMAL OPENING

SLIGHT CLOSING

MARKED
NARROWING

HARDENING OF
THE ARTERIES

The above illustration shows the silting up process in the coronary arteries which supply the heart with blood. This process is called arteriosclerosis, or hardening of the arteries.

It is in these narrowed blood vessels that a blood clot blocks the flow of blood, causing coronary occlusion, with angina pectoris pains, commonly referred to as a 'heart attack'.

2

Coronary Heart Disease

Whilst coronary heart disease is the leading cause of death in Britain and other Western countries it is only one-tenth as common in industrial Japan and rare in most Third World communities. However, once immigrant groups leave these countries for the West their incidence of coronary heart disease approaches that of their host country in a generation or two. It is a relatively recent disease, since it was uncommon before 1925 but then its incidence rose steadily except for a dip in Europe during the second world war. Coronary heart disease is now declining in the USA and Australia, is static in Britain and most of Western Europe but is steadily increasing in Eastern Europe.

Finland holds the doubtful pride of place in the deaths from coronary heart disease league in the figures for 1978, taken from the National Heart Foundation of New Zealand—Coronary Heart Disease, Auckland and the National Heart Foundation (UK) in 1983. The tragic figures are (per 100,000 population in the forty-five to fifty age range) Finland 441; Scotland 432; USA 339; England and Wales 322; Australia and New Zealand 300; Sweden 186; Greece 116; Japan 35.

What are the reasons for coronary heart disease?
There are many factors that can contribute to the chances of getting coronary heart disease but it is now becoming

generally accepted that diet is probably the fundamental environmental one that we can control. What we eat can determine the process of atherosclerosis which takes years to develop; our food can cause a thrombosis to be deposited on the atherosclerotic plaque which can happen in hours and the diet can give rise to changes in the ECG. All three processes can be factors in the fatal heart attack, in the development of angina or weakening of the heart muscle. Before we consider the role of diet in detail, let us look at other risk factors that can contribute to the chances of our having coronary heart disease.

Family pattern: There is no doubt that a tendency to develop coronary heart disease runs in certain families. If your parents, aunts and uncles, brothers and sisters have had problems with the heart, you stand a greater risk of developing heart complaints yourself than if your close relatives lived to a ripe old age with trouble-free hearts. On the other hand it does not follow that you will necessarily have heart problems even if they did nor does lack of heart disease in your immediate family exempt you from the possibilities of developing it. In either case however, careful control of your diet and other risk factors can reduce your chances of succumbing to a heart complaint. You cannot alter hereditary tendencies but all other factors are in your hands.

Weight watching: There is no doubt that many fat people enjoy excellent health and die in their seventies and eighties. Perhaps this reflects their easy going, good humoured and benevolent natures but in the cold world of economics such individuals are regarded by Life Assurance companies as bad risks. In general, lean people are less prone to illness than fat ones and because post-operative complications are commoner in the obese, surgeons do not like operating on them.

Excessive weight can cause an increase in blood-pressure—recent studies indicate that a small rise can be reversed simply by reducing weight—and a high blood-pressure (hypertension) is one of the most important factors in increasing the chances of coronary heart disease. We shall discuss this later on. In addition though, obesity can aggravate arthritis in hips and knees because of the extra weight on the load-bearing joints of the body.

You must therefore avoid putting on extra weight and this factor of course can in most cases be controlled completely by sensible eating. As well as making you feel and look healthier and younger, keeping your weight down will also help protect your heart. Find your ideal weight, from one of the many tables published, for your age, sex and height and try to stick with it. For every 20 lb overweight your diastolic blood-pressure (the lower one your doctor measures) will increase by at least 3mm mercury. Conversely, a 10 lb weight loss can reduce the diastolic blood-pressure by at least 5mm mercury (the higher systolic pressure reduces by 10mm).

As well as increasing the blood-pressure, recent long-term studies (including the Framingham Heart Study which followed individuals over twenty-six years) suggest that there is a positive correlation between blood cholesterol and body weight.

Another study called the Zutphen Study (named after the small Netherlands town in which it was conducted for more than twenty years starting in 1960) was carried out on randomly selected men in the forty to fifty-nine age range. It was found that average blood cholesterol levels increased significantly with increased body weight. A rise of only 2.2 lbs (1kg) was associated with a 2mg rise in blood cholesterol. Conversely, a reduction in weight would be expected to reduce the blood cholesterol by a similar amount presumably by a decreased intake of fatty, cholesterol-containing foods. The study concluded 'In a free-living, weight-gaining population of middle-aged men, body weight is the most important determinant of serum cholesterol. Evidence is also accumulating that in such a population dietary cholesterol is a determinant of serum cholesterol independent of body weight.'

Smoking tobacco: There is now overwhelming evidence that smoking tobacco is a major factor in the development of coronary heart disease. Reducing or giving up the habit completely greatly diminishes the danger. The risk of dying from coronary heart disease appears to be at least twice as great in smokers as in non-smokers. A study of British doctors (who should have known better) revealed that those who smoked tabocco had between four and five times the frequency of death from coronary heart disease than their non-smoking colleagues between the ages of thirty-five and fifty-four.

No one is quite sure of the precise way in which tobacco smoke causes or aggravates disease of the coronary and other arteries but two smoke constituents have been implicated. One is nicotine that adversely affects the functioning of the heart and arteries. The other, carbon monoxide, is a poison that works by replacing oxygen that is usually carried by the haemoglobin of the red blood cells. Carbon monoxide deprives the blood of the life-giving oxygen and so depletes the heart muscle of this essential nutrient. It is also significant that the constituents of tobacco smoke can destroy certain essential components of heart muscle cells such as vitamins B_1 and C and the essential sulphur-containing amino acids. Local deficiency of these micronutrients can induce unwelcome changes in the metabolism of heart muscle with subsequent increased chances of disease developing. The soundest advice, however, is simple. Do not smoke.

Exercise: As our way of life and work has become progressively mechanized so everyday exercise has steadily decreased in the main sector of the population. Where once people walked or cycled to work, they now ride. Urbanization has reduced the open spaces where games could be organized. Television encourages relaxation rather than exercise so the required balance is geared towards sitting rather than doing something. At the same time the percentage of the population whose occupation requires more than light physical exertion is on the decrease. The introduction of excavators and tractors whilst essential in modern working conditions has meant less physical effort by the navvy and the farmer.

Our way of life now means that most of us can get through the day with a walk of half-a-mile at the most and too often this is the only daily exercise. The question immediately arises: 'What is the amount of exercise we need to prevent a heart attack?' This is impossible to assess because no one can state dogmatically that lack of exercise is an important factor in the development of coronary heart disease. What is certain is that it must play some part because the incidence of the disease is less in those with physically active occupations.

Despite popular belief, it is safe to say that no amount of physical activity will harm a healthy person. The body will adapt to countless forms of exertion and it does demand exercise. This is not to say that anyone can run a marathon because like any supreme effort such an activity requires training to adapt the unfit body to the unaccustomed exercise. What it is looking for is walking, golf, swimming, gardening at one end of the scale to the more intense jogging, squash, tennis and badminton at the other. These are exertions that can be carried out throughout the year where age represents no barrier. If pursued at least twice a week these exercises are likely to reduce, at least to some extent, your chances of developing a heart ailment.

How does exercise help to ward off heart attacks? One answer may be in the relationship that has been found between exercise and blood cholesterol levels. This connection has been observed at two levels of exercise, vigorous and moderate. Although in the past it was asserted that only high-level exercise like competitive swimming, long-distance running or cross-country skiing were beneficial, recent studies suggest otherwise.

The Australian National University Mountaineering Club organized an eight-week climb in the Himalayas for thirteen of their members from the ages of twenty-two to forty-three. The men were monitored closely in terms of body weight, smoking and food intake. Alcohol intake was zero in all of them. Body weight was constant despite an increased intake of starches and sugar. It was obvious that the strenuous exercise undergone could balance out the increased calories but the most important finding was that their blood cholesterol levels all became normal with an increased proportion of the protective HDL-cholesterol (see later). Of course, the intense cold, high altitude and reduced oxygen concentration in the rarefied air may have contributed but the results confirmed those noted in other studies when cholesterol levels after intense exercise were measured.

Exercise need not be so strenuous and studies at the Laboratory of Physiological Hygiene of the University of Minnesota's School of Public Health confirmed that cholesterol can be controlled even on moderate exercise. The studies were performed on sedentary middle-aged men and the criteria measured were body weight, blood fats, blood cholesterol and skinfold thickness, which gives an indication of body fat. All were on a fat-controlled diet. Exercise consisted simply of an hour walking on a treadmill three times a week at an average speed of 3 miles per hour on a 4 per cent uphill grade. The control group did no walking.

After twelve weeks of this, the men who had exercised lost more weight and body fat than those who had not. The blood levels of cholesterol and types of cholesterol were also more favourable in the walkers. Hence even this mild exercise regime when carried out on a regular basis results in benefits that can cut down the chances of developing a heart attack. Exercise is no guarantee against death from sudden heart attacks but it can be invigorating and possibly life-extending for all.

High blood-pressure: Maintaining blood-pressure is a result of the heart's pumping action and the elasticity of the arteries. This pumping action is essential to distribute blood to all the parts of the body that needs it and if the heart slows or even stops beating the blood-pressure goes very low or falls to zero and blood ceases to circulate. This is why those with persistent low blood-pressure may have a desirable condition from their cardiologists point of view but they can still suffer when the blood supply to the brain and other extremities is curtailed.

Blood-pressure in anyone is a variable entity changing from moment to moment depending upon our state of physical and mental activity. There is no fixed figure or upper limit that will apply to everyone but there is a normal range and it is when this is exceeded by a significant amount that it is possible to say that you suffer from raised blood-pressure or hypertension. The pressure rises because the heart has to work harder to pump against what is usually a constricted set of arteries. At the same time it must pump against the high pressure created in the arteries so a vicious circle sets in. One constricted main artery will cause high blood-pressure in all of them.

As this state of affairs continues both heart and arteries will suffer. The heart gets bigger and eventually may fail, and the constant high pressure on the arteries increases wear and tear on them just as pipes suffer when subjected to high-pressure liquids or steam. When the blood-pressure is consistently high, the blood vessels in the brain are prone to collapse or burst resulting in a stroke. At the same time heart attacks are far more likely in those with high blood-pressure.

Whilst control of the blood-pressure by weight reduction or medicinal drugs has been proved to reduce the likelihood of strokes and heart failure there is no convincing evidence that it will prevent heart attacks in those with existing coronary heart disease. What you can do, however, is help yourself to reduce the chances of heart disease by dietary approaches first through prevention but even in a pre-existing condition further deterioration can be halted by control of the diet and sensible supplementation. Such approaches can complement conventional medical treatment also.

Stress and anxiety: It is difficult to evaluate the part played by mental stress in the development of coronary heart disease. Objective evidence of a direct relationship is very hard to find. Nevertheless, since the mental states of anxiety, fear, irritation and frustration are unpleasant there is much to be said for avoiding them if you can. There is no doubt that avoidance may mean a change of occupation; shedding of one's commitments, solving a domestic problem or, if you are lucky, simply adapting to a more philosophical attitude of life. Do not duck out of every challenge but try to pinpoint the cause of your stress and anxiety and if you cannot do anything about it yourself, look elsewhere for help or change your lifestyle.

It is generally accepted that stress can raise blood cholesterol levels but just how much is difficult to quantify. The high cholesterol may be one factor in the role of stress as a major coronary heart disease risk but it is related also to other risk factors such as high blood-pressure, overeating, smoking, alcohol and drug abuse and of course inherited personality traits. Let us look at how the type of person you are may influence your susceptibility to heart attacks.

The personality category known as type A is usually regarded as being especially vulnerable to stress and heart attacks. The behaviour of these people is characterized by feelings of urgency about time, where they hate to be kept waiting and feel that everything is rush, rush, rush. These individuals ignore advice from friends and family to slow down; they will not wait for others to complete their say; they speak rapidly; they blink frequently; they clench fists and will pound desk or table. They will eat quickly and often compulsively. In all walks of life, these people are fiercely competitive and impatient of obstacles that stand in the way of ambition.

Type-A behaviour can however be modified, even after it may have led to a heart attack. These people can avoid a recurrence by bringing under control their stressful, aggressive way of relating to others. One study carried out at the Mount Zion Hospital and Medical Centre in San Francisco and Stanford University School of Medicine was on 800 men of type A who had suffered a heart attack. Once they were encouraged and helped to curb their sense of urgency, their competitiveness, their inability to relax and their easily aroused frustration, suspicion and hostility, their chances of a second heart attack were reduced. In this group there were only 50 per cent of the expected second heart attacks.

Perhaps the simplest approach is that suggested by Dr Herbert Benson, who called it the Relaxation Response. It can be used by anyone but is particularly suited to type A people and those undergoing any kind of stress. Each morning and evening the individual sits quietly for ten to fifteen minutes with the eyes closed, repeating with each breath a simple, single syllable.

Special cases: There are two types of people who because of their condition or because of what they are taking appear to have an increased chance of developing coronary heart disease. The first is those who suffer from diabetes.

Diabetes is a disorder of body chemistry where for one reason or another, the muscles are unable to take up glucose from the blood. Certain cells in the pancreas, a gland situated just behind the stomach with its head attached to the duodenum and its tail reaching to the spleen, produce a hormone called insulin. Insulin has the specific function of controlling the handling of glucose within the body. Hence when it is lacking, blood sugar levels tend to be higher than normal and this leads to certain complications within the body metabolism. Diabetes develops when insulin is no longer secreted by the pancreas or when its production is diminished. It is also possible to have diabetes when the hormone is secreted but is not utilized as it should be. Whilst there is no evidence that diabetes itself contributes to the higher frequency of coronary heart disease prevalent in diabetics, there is no doubt that those with the disease have a greater chance of developing heart problems. Diabetics are subject to other risk factors that may also be important. What is of interest, however, is that diabetics may be more prone to specific deficiencies of some vitamins and minerals because of their condition and these deficiencies may give rise to the later manifestations of the disease. The dietary advice given in this book to ward off and perhaps even treat coronary heart disease applies equally well to those suffering from diabetes.

The second sector of the population who should be concerned about coronary heart disease because of what they are taking are those women on the contraceptive pill. During the almost thirty years that the effects of this form of contraception have been studied, it has been noted that women over forty taking the pill have an increased risk of heart attack compared with those not taking the preparation. It must be said, however, that other risk factors such as heavy smoking appear to potentiate the effects of the pill constituents. In some women the pill is associated with high blood-pressure and even on rare occasions with strokes.

Happily, it does look as if younger women who are healthy and do not smoke have less to worry about the complications of the pill than their older colleagues. In fact the risks are so small that the benefits of oral contraception outweigh any disadvantages. However, once a women reaches over the age of thirty-five, she should be aware that the constituents of the contraceptive pill may increase her chances of coronary heart disease and she should seek professional advice before continuing with this type of contraception.

The causes of coronary heart disease discussed above are all of non-dietary origin and there is no doubt that they do contribute to increasing the chances of developing the complaint. However, it now appears that even more important than these causes is that of wrong diet and this is something that is entirely under our own control. Let us now look at how dietary factors can contribute to our chances of getting coronary heart disease. First and foremost must be cholesterol and fat intakes and even more importantly their levels within the body.

Cholesterol: Cholesterol is a fatty substance that is present in significant amounts only in fats of animal, fowl and fish origin. Hence whilst those who eat these foods obtain some from their diet, much of our body cholesterol comes by synthesis from within. Vegetarians obtain some from the dairy products they may eat; vegans obtain virtually none from their diet. In the normal, healthy person, an increased dietary intake of cholesterol is tempered by a decreased synthesis within the body and vice versa. In this way, normal blood cholesterol levels are maintained but too often, excessive dietary intakes or increased synthesis within the body will give rise to high blood levels. We can reduce our dietary intake easily but even when body synthesis is too high, we can do much to control it by dietary means. If these are not undertaken then powerful drugs must be used.

Cholesterol is essential to our health as it contributes to at least three valuable functions within the body. It is a constituent of cell membranes, particularly the myelin sheath that insulates nerves; it is a precursor of the bile acids that are needed to help emulsify fats before they can be digested; it is needed as a precursor of steroid hormones that control sexual function, water balance, stress and metabolic actions. A derivative of cholesterol called 7-dehydrocholesterol is produced in the skin where it is acted upon by ultra-violet light to supply us with vitamin D. Blood plasma cholesterol levels of healthy adults range widely in different communities from 120mg per 100ml (3 millimoles per litre) in Bushmen and Nasai to 280mg per 100ml (7.2 millimoles per litre) in Finland. In Britain and the West generally, average total blood plasma cholesterol exceeds 200mg per 100ml (5.2 millimoles per litre). It is highly significant that only in those countries where this figure is exceeded is coronary heart disease common. These are simply population observations but recently the relationship between high blood plasma levels and the development of coronary heart disease was proved on a firmer basis.

In 1984, the National Heart, Lung and Blood Institute

in the USA announced the results of a comprehensive study to determine whether lowering blood cholesterol would decrease the incidence of heart disease. For more than ten years, almost 4,000 men had been monitored in a double blind investigation, i.e. neither subjects nor investigators knew who was receiving special treatment. Only men between thirty-five and fifty-nine years were studied at the outset, and all had blood plasma levels of cholesterol in excess of 265mg per 100ml. All restricted their dietary intakes of cholesterol to 400mg daily but one-half of them received a cholesterol lowering drug in addition. Some were controlled by diet alone.

The results justified any measures, either drug or diet, that culminated in a reduction in blood cholesterol. The risk of heart attack deaths was found to drop 2 per cent for every 1 per cent reduction in blood cholesterol. It did not matter whether the cholesterol was lowered by medication alone, diet alone or a mixture of the two. A reduced blood cholesterol lowered the chances of coronary heart disease.

The originators of the trial concluded that the average blood cholesterol levels of adults between 200 and 230mg per 100ml were too high. Anyone over the age of thirty should have a reading of 200mg or less. Any level above 200mg places the individual in a moderate to high risk of a heart attack. We should all strive to get our cholesterol levels down to those observed in the populations of countries like Japan, Greece and almost all non-Westernized countries where coronary heart disease is rare. We shall see later how we can adapt our diet to reach this desirable goal.

Types of cholesterol carriers

Although high-blood levels of cholesterol are considered undesirable, research over the last few years has indicated that the way in which cholesterol is carried in the blood is an important factor in determining the chances of a heart attack. Cholesterol is a waxy substance that is insoluble in water so it can move through the bloodstream only on the back of specific proteins called lipoproteins. These lipoproteins are four in number but only in three of them are significant amounts of cholesterol carried in the blood. They all differ in their bulkiness or density.

Chylomicrons are the largest lipoproteins. They are about 80 to 95 per cent fat with only small amounts of cholesterol, protein and particular type of fat called phospholipid (lecithin is a good example of a phospholipid). Chylomicrons carry the fat from the food you eat through the intestines into the blood-stream. They all end up in the liver where the fatty part is burned off as energy to make new cells and produce heat. Any left over are stored in the cells for later energy production but obviously over-storage is undesirable and will eventually affect the workings of the liver. Lecithin is one natural phospholipid that prevents this happening. Chylomicrons, however, play little part in carrying cholesterol once they are absorbed from the food.

VLDL or *very low-density lipoproteins* are mostly fat (60 to 80 per cent) but they do not come from the food. Instead they are manufactured by the liver. Their main function is to carry the fats synthesized by the liver to the fatty tissues of the body, via the bloodstream, so that fat (or energy) reserves can be built up. Any leftovers are simply transported back to the liver which uses them to make more fats. VLDL are hence used in a recycling-type process. They carry some cholesterol but not significant amounts.

LDL or *low-density lipoprotein* is the dangerous one, being responsible for carrying between 50 and 60 per cent of the blood's total cholesterol content. It also supplies the cholesterol that is deposited on the inside of blood vessel walls and so contributing to the constriction of them. LDL consists mainly of cholesterol with only about 25 per cent protein. Hence it has a special transportation problem because although it can enter an artery, it cannot easily get out. Once trapped, the LDL breaks down, liberating the waxy cholesterol to be deposited on the walls of the blood vessel. Once this happens, the way is clear for the gradual built up of fat in the blood vessel that we call atherosclerosis.

HDL or *high-density lipoprotein* is the good carrier of cholesterol. It is mostly protein with some phospholipid but contains only a small to moderate amount of cholesterol along with very little fat. It functions by removing harmful fats like LDL cholesterol from the blood and from the walls of the arteries. HDL acts like a detergent and hence is a good protective force against fat and cholesterol being deposited in the wrong places.

We need all these different types of lipoprotein carrying cholesterol and fats so the prime objective to stay healthy is to maintain the correct balance of them all. The ideal situation therefore is to increase the level of protective HDL cholesterol and reduce the quality of destructive LDL cholesterol. It is no longer sufficient to talk simply of cholesterol levels in the blood, we must also know that we have the right sort of cholesterol in the blood, namely HDL cholesterol. As we shall see, the easiest way to do this is by dietary means. Once our blood cholesterol levels are down to normal and they are in the right form, we have diminished our chances of having a heart attack in one risk factor at least.

The situation has been summed up neatly by Dr Simeon Margolis of the Johns Hopkins School of Medicine who wrote in April 1981: 'Levels of serum cholesterol carried mainly on low-density lipoproteins (LDL) correlate strongly with the development of myocardial infarction (heart attack). In contrast, considerable evidence indicates that high-density liprotein (HDL) protects against coronary heart disease.'

3

Other Heart Complaints

Let us now look at some of the other heart complaints and their symptoms. As we shall see, some of the milder symptoms we may notice have no significance whatsoever and are simply a feature of the complex workings of the heart. On the other hand, if any of these symptoms occur regularly or persist, professional advice should be sought so that heart disease as a cause may be eliminated.

Angina
Although not strictly a heart complaint, angina pectoris is the commonest early symptom of coronary artery disease. It literally means 'pain of the breast'. It is a tight, constricting or band-like sensation, usually felt across the middle of the chest. Sometimes it spreads to the armpits, down the arms or to the neck or jaw and occasionally to the back between the shoulder blades. It can vary from a mild discomfort to a severe pain.

The symptom characteristically comes on when the work of the heart is increased by exercise or even by emotion. It is more often provoked in cold weather or when exercising after meals. Sometimes the hasty eating of a meal, the eating of too much food, sudden over-exertion or intense excitement are enough to provoke an attack. Since it may happen after meals, many sufferers imagine they have indigestion and take the appropriate medicine which of course has no beneficial effect upon the angina.

The pain of angina arises in the heart muscle and is a result of narrowing in one or more of the coronary arteries which reduces the blood supply to the heart and hence deprives it of oxygen. As well as not receiving enough oxygen there is a slowing down of the removal of waste products from the heart muscle because this process also requires an adequate blood supply. The accumulation of these waste products stimulates nerve endings and causes the pain. Angina can therefore be regarded as heart cramp or heart pang. A similar condition can arise in the leg when the arteries are constricted and the individual experiences pain in the calves or thighs when they work too far or too fast. This complaint is known as intermittent claudication.

Breathlessness

Most of those suffering from angina also complain of shortness of breath when their attack comes on. This is because the left ventricle, which does the pumping of the blood to the body, cannot function efficiently when short of oxygen. Consequently, pressure of blood builds up behind it as oxygenated blood is supplied from the lungs. Lack of clearance of blood from the lungs causes congestion in those organs and there is a sensation of laboured breathing. Even when angina is absent, some may experience only abnormal breathlessness when they exercise.

Palpitating hearts

Although palpitating and thumping hearts are common in heart disease, they happen almost as often in those with healthy hearts and can make these people believe they have a heart complaint. Palpitation can thus arise from an awareness of abnormal heart function or from an abnormal awareness of normal heart function. Anyone who focuses attention on his or her chest will feel or even hear their heart thumping after sharp exercise or before a test, audition or interview. This is a perfectly normal reaction and simply reflects mild anxiety. Similarly it is not difficult to feel your heart beating when lying in certain positions in bed—the mattress can often act as a sounding board. However, in all these circumstances the action and rhythm of the heart are normal even though its beat may appear to be fast or heavy.

Extra heartbeats

The heart is such a magnificent organ with such superb control that it is able to beat regularly for hours yet accelerate when called upon to do so and at the other end of the scale it can slow down when we are at rest or asleep. Nevertheless, irregularities of the beat do occur and if we are monitored continuously enough it is likely we could all pick up an extra beat or so over the day.

The commonest event is an extra beat occurring just a little before its proper time and followed by a pause before the next beat follows. Usually the individual is unaware of the early or premature beat which is not very strong because the heart has had less time to fill. What is noticed is the beat after the pause which is stronger because in this case the heart has had longer to fill and so pumps out more blood. The beat gives a sensation of a thump or thud in the chest and it is often described as 'missing a beat'. This event occurs in all of us from time to time and is of no consequence in a healthy person but it can engender unnecessary anxiety if an individual is at all nervous about their state of health.

Rapid heartbeats

The extra beats described above are much more common in coronary heart disease and may be a symptom of abnormal heart function. What can happen is that the normal 'pacemaker' of the heart loses control and the heart starts racing fast or very fast indeed. This sort of rhythm disturbance is important and merits medical advice and attention. It is easily detected on the ECG. Much less commonly we see the other extreme where the heart beats too slowly. In this case, the individual is less aware of a slow heartbeat but is more likely to complain of its manifestations including undue fatigue, light-headedness, dizziness and perhaps even blackouts.

Dizziness

This, along with faintness, is common and like palpitation frequently has nothing at all to do with heart disease or any other physical disorder. There are occasions, however, when such symptoms are important and point to abnormal heart rhythm, anaemia or low blood-pressure. Whether beating too fast or too slowly, the heart is at a mechanical disadvantage and will not pump out the desired volume of blood. This state of affairs is not signalled by most organs of the body but the brain is the exception. It objects within a few seconds to any shortage of its blood and hence oxygen supply and if deprived too long, loss of consciousness will occur. For this reason, any faintness or dizziness may be important and should be reported to your practitioner.

Anxiety

It is regrettable but true that anxiety can produce changes in body function that resemble those that are symptomatic of organic disease. We have seen that dizziness, chest pain and palpitation can occur in the absence of heart disease. Chest pains for example, can be explained by spasm or cramp in one of the small muscles between the ribs. The more sudden the onset of pain the less likelihood that it is connected with a heart complaint.

It is not uncommon for an individual who suffers from

such an innocent pain to respond by breathing deeply and rapidly. This is known as hyperventilation and whilst appropriate after a burst of exercise is not to be recommended at rest. It leads to widespread body changes caused by the blowing out from the lungs of excess amounts of carbon dioxide. This in turn induces dizziness, tight feelings in the chest and tingling in the face and extremities. Hence a natural response to one worry leads to even more worrisome symptoms. Again, if these occur often it is sensible to report them to your doctor who can eliminate heart disease as contributing to them. It is surprising how often simple reassurance is the most effective way to remove such symptoms.

We have seen that true angina needs correct diagnosis by a medical practitioner but at the same time many of its symptoms can be due to causes other than coronary heart disease. Let us now consider some of the other heart conditions that may arise, which also need confirmation of diagnosis by a professional before drug therapy is instituted. Later we shall see how dietary measures can often prevent such heart complaints from arising but even when they have been diagnosed, such complaints should also be treated by dietary means which complement (but not replace) any drug treatment that is given.

Hypertrophy

Hypertrophy of the heart: This condition is often developed by people submitting the heart to abnormal strain, such as athletes. The heart becomes enlarged. Behind this condition, however, there is usually a history of wrong feeding and the slow poisoning of the blood-stream. One authority says: 'Where there is hypertrophy, it means that in attempting to carry on its full activities under a condition of great strain, one or both of the lower ventricles of the heart have become enlarged to enable it to cope with the abnormal task.' Some people with enlarged hearts suffer little inconvenience, but with others the condition is accompanied by dizziness, headache and head noises.

Dilatation of the heart: This is usually a development of hypertrophy. It means that the compensating factors of heart enlargement have deteriorated. Dilatation is a condition of decided weakness and danger. Shortness of breath after the slightest exertion, disturbed sleep, more or less continual discomfort in the region of the heart, palpitation, etc., are its accompanying symptoms.

Endocarditis, myocarditis and pericarditis

Endocarditis: This is a condition in which there is inflammation of the membrane which lines the cavities of the heart. The disease may be acute, or chronic, and is positively associated with a highly toxic condition of the system. Endocarditis usually leads to definite disease of the heart.

Myocarditis: This is the term used to denote inflammation of the muscular tissue of the heart. The condition may be acute or chronic and leads to progressive degeneration of the heart muscle with greater or lesser impairment of heart action.

Pericarditis: This is the term applied to inflammation of the pericardium, or membranous sac in which the heart is enclosed.

Anaemia and the heart

Blood is red because of floating red discs called red blood

cells. They contain a subtance (haemoglobin) that carries oxygen from the lungs to the heart muscle and other body tissues. One may think of them as rail-road cars. They carry their product (oxygen) from the point of supply (lungs) to the consumer (heart muscle). If these red cells become fewer and fewer for any one of many causes, a condition called anaemia is present. This means that even though there is an adequate supply of oxygen in the lungs, there are not enough rail-road cars (red cells) to carry it to the consumer (heart muscle). If such a state is allowed to continue, the heart suffers.

Valvular diseases

Valvular disease of the heart may be of various kinds, ranging in degree from very serious to comparatively slight. In valvular heart disease the valves which shut off the heart chambers one from another, or which shut off the great arteries leading from the heart itself, have become either too large or too small, thus interferring with the proper passage of the blood to and from the heart, with greater or lesser disturbance of bodily function. The greater predisposing factor towards the setting up of valvular heart disease is inflammation of the heart lining (endocarditis); and this is often the outcome of rheumatic fever, scarlet fever, etc., plus a blood-stream systematically poisoned over a period of years — a heart muscle starved of vitamin E.

Congestive heart failure

When the heart muscle becomes weakened, overfatigued or 'strained' and can no longer meet the demands made upon it, a condition known as congestive heart failure exists. For example, in cases of high blood-pressure in which the heart is enlarged to the limit of its coronary blood supply, the cardiac reserve is used up and the heart is no longer an efficient pump, the following things happen as a result. The left ventricle is tired and can no longer completely empty the pumping chamber. A small amount of blood remains in the ventricle after contraction. The left auricle contracts, but because of the blood already in the ventricle it cannot completely empty itself. Blood backs up and produces congestion in the lungs. The right ventricle cannot empty, the left auricle cannot empty, and the blood backs up in the tissues. Because of the back pressure in the veins carrying blood right back to the heart, fluid from the blood leaks out into the tissues and causes swelling. The ankles and legs are the first to show this swelling known as dropsy or oedema. The patient with congestive heart failure complains of shortness of breath and he may develop an irritating cough because of the congestion in his lungs. The veins of his neck may stand out, and his ankles become swollen. All these symptoms may result from a tired and inefficient central pumping system.

Other heart ailments

Mitral stenosis: A constriction or narrowing of the mitral valve between the left auricle and left ventricle.

Bradycardia: A slowness of the heartbeat with a rhythm of less than fifty beats a minutes.

Tachycardia: Excessive rapidity of the heart's action, with a rhythm exceeding one hundred beats a minute.

Early symptoms of heart trouble
The following are the symptoms which indicate that you may be heading for heart trouble:
(1) Breathlessness upon such exertions as going up stairs

or steps, hurrying for a train, etc., and/or a feeling of fatigue or exhaustion following any undue exertion.

(2) Discomfort in sleeping. A desire to prop oneself up in bed so that one may breathe more freely.

(3) Giddiness or light-headedness.

(4) A sensation of dull pressure on the breastbone, extending to the left shoulder and down the left arm. In some cases only the left shoulder and arm may be affected.

(5) Pains in the chest after meals, or upon exertion. These are often taken for indigestion pains, when they are angina symptoms.

A person may experience no more than one or two of those symptoms, but he should take them as definite warnings that more serious heart trouble is ahead if prompt steps are not taken to:

(a) Strengthen the heart muscle with a moderate amount of vitamin E daily;

(b) Improve the general nervous system and the nerves of the heart with B complex vitamin tablets daily;

(c) Reduce the viscosity of the blood by eating much less meat and egg proteins;

(d) Reduce the deposit of cholesterol in the arteries by cutting down on all fat foods;

(e) Cut down on sugary and sweetened foods and drinks.

(f) Build up the general health by sound nutrition as advocated further on in this book.

More serious symptoms of heart trouble

The following are symptoms of heart trouble of a more advanced nature:

(1) Breathlessness upon exertion and a sense of fatigue or exhaustion after it.

(2) Racing heart (tachycardia).

(3) Pain in the region of the breastbone. It may be slight,

but in a 'heart attack', it is usually agonizing and alarming, spreading down the left arm, and accompanied by a painful choking constriction in the chest, and a state of collapse. These are the symptoms of the dreaded angina pectoris, commonly referred to as a 'heart attack'.

(4) Swellings in the ankles and feet. This dropsical condition is called oedema. The tissues of the ankles and feet become saturated with fluid. This is a sign of congestive heart failure.

(5) In congestive heart failure fluid can also seep into the lungs, causing shortness of breath, congestion of the lungs and irritating cough.

What is a heart attack?

There is much confusion amongst people as to exactly what is meant by a heart attack. The popular expression 'he's had a coronary' is more meaningful because coronary is short for coronary thrombosis. It means a blood clot has formed which obstructs a coronary artery. In more exacting terms 'heart attack' or 'coronary' should mean that actual damage to the heart muscle has occurred as the result of impaired or interrupted blood flow to a part of the main pumping chamber or left ventricle. Proof of damage can come only from ECG and by the measurement of certain enzymes released into the blood from the injured muscle.

The medical term for heart attack is 'Myocardial Infarction' which means that a portion of the heart muscle has been destroyed by deprivation of its blood supply. Usually this is because a narrowed artery has been blocked with a blood clot but it can also arise because the blood supply through diseased arteries has been reduced for some other reason. The main symptom is a pain similar to but more severe than the average attack of angina but in addition there are often other symptoms like sweating or vomiting.

Anyone who suffers from angina may therefore pass off the anginal pain as just another attack of angina but the sweating and vomiting suggest a more severe one. Some may also experience breathlessness and faintness during an attack which can occasionally lead to unconsciousness. When possible the sufferer should place himself in a reclining chair or lie down in bed in whichever position he finds most comfortable and await professional help. Self-treatment with anti-angina drugs is unlikely to be of much use in an actual heart attack but if the pain is relieved this is a good sign. The unpleasant symptoms can persist for any time from an hour to a couple of days.

During the early phases of a heart attack there is a disturbance in heart rhythm. This complication may have little effect on the pumping action of the heart but sometimes there may be an arrest of the blood circulation which is serious. If this happens the only thing the untrained person can do is to stimulate the heart by striking the chest wall below the left nipple with a clenched fist hard enough to cause a bruise.

Failure to stimulate the heart in this manner means that heart massage must be attempted. This involves compressing the heart between breast bone and spine about once a second by firm downward movement of the hands which are placed one on top of each other over the lower heart of the breast bone. This action squeezes blood out of the heart and can maintain circulation until the heart starts up again.

If breathing has stopped, it is necessary to give the 'kiss of life'. It means blowing air into the person's mouth to ventilate his lungs and hence stimulate his own breathing reflex. Often this is not necessary if external heart massage is started within half-a-minute of the circulatory arrest. Nothing else can be attempted until professional help arrives.

It is important to realize that an attack of angina is not

a heart attack or coronary because there is no destruction of heart muscle. A prolonged anginal attack may be mistaken for a heart attack but only the heart specialist can detect any actual death of an area of heart muscle. Once this has happened it is important to assess the extent of the damage. The heart has great reserves of power and a small affected area is unlikely to affect its functioning too much.

The portion of muscle that has died because its oxygen supply has stopped gradually shrinks and is replaced by fibrous or scar tissue. The whole process takes about six weeks and it is during this critical period that the heart must be protected from excessive work.

Drug therapy of heart complaints

Digitalis: The oldest established heart drug used today is digitalis, a natural substance extracted from the common foxglove flower. It is known as a cardiac glycoside and it functions by increasing the force of contraction of the heart without increasing its oxygen consumption. It is therefore used when the heart-pumping action is weak as in heart failure. Unfortunately, however, digitalis and other cardiac glycosides have little effect upon the heart until they are present in potencies near those at which toxic effects occur. It is necessary therefore that the dosage is carefully controlled. The usual dosage regime is to start with high potency then reduce to a low potency that maintains the concentration of the drug at that required to replace its daily losses. This process is called digitalization.

Side effects are common because the margin between effective and toxic doses is small. Nausea, salivation, vomiting and loss of appetite are amongst the earliest symptoms of digitalis overdosage. Diarrhoea and abdominal pain may also occur. There are also headache, facial pain, malaise, drowsiness, depression, mental confusion, and tingling and numbness in the hands and feet. The eyes are affected by blurred vision and there may be a disturbance of colour vision. Irregular heartbeats are also a sign of overdosage. Side-effects are exacerbated by depletion of potassium induced by diuretic drugs.

Coronary vasodilators

These drugs are used chiefly for the prevention and treatment of angina because they dilate the blood vessels, lower blood-pressure and reduce the work of the heart. A typical drug is glyceryl trinitrate which is sucked or chewed when the pain happens. The active substance is absorbed from the mouth and is useless if swallowed. Usually no more than one should be taken at a time or at intervals shorter than twenty minutes. These drugs are taken only by those suffering from angina.

Possible side-effects are flushing of the face, dizziness, tachycardia (fast heartbeat) and throbbing headache. Large doses can cause vomiting, restlessness, low blood-pressure, fainting and blood problems. Coldness of the skin with impairment of respiration can also happen.

Beta-blocking drugs

The drugs are in common use in the treatment of angina. They function by interfering with or blocking the stimulation of the heart by the nerves that supply it. Hence they reduce the rate and force of contraction of the heart and by decreasing the rate of conduction of electrical impulses through the conducting system, the response of the heart to stress and exercise is reduced. The net result is a reduction of oxygen consumption by heart muscle and so the drugs also increase the tolerance of the heart to exercise. Although developed essentially for angina treatment, betablockers can also be used to treat irregular heartbeats. They are used to reduce high blood-pressure but their mode of action here is unknown. Recently the drugs have been found to be of benefit in mild anxiety conditions like those that occur before examinations and auditions.

The most common side-effects are nausea, vomiting, diarrhoea, fatigue and dizziness. Effects on the heart include slowing of the heart rate, low blood-pressure and sometimes heart failure. Cold extremities are often the result of beta-blocker treatment. Constipation, weight gain, muscle cramps and dry mouth are not uncommon.

Why the usual treatment fails

If you are a sufferer from some heart ailment it won't help you a scrap to be told that you suffer from, say, endocarditis instead of say, myocarditis. These shades of difference in heart ailments interest the medical profession, but they are of little significance to the sufferer. Why do we say that? Because all these fine distinctions in heart disaffection are merely different manifestations of the same causation. If you are interested in removing the trouble you will naturally look to the factors that have caused it, and having once ascertained them, you will discontinue those practices or habits. That is the simple, commonsense action to take.

But how does the average orthodox doctor proceed to treat the heart sufferer? Chiefly by rest and the use of drugs. The most dangerous weapon in the armoury of orthodox medicine is its reliance upon drugs to effect a cure, whether it be the heart or any other organ. The specialist who uses digitalis to slow the rapid heart, adrenalin to accelerate a slow heart, amyl nitrate to relax a tense heart, or trinitrite to dilate a restricted artery, has succeeded at best in stopping a symptom, temporarily, by imposing great additional strains upon an already over-loaded organ and its controls.

The following extract from Dr W. H. Gordon's book on the heart—Dr Gordon is one of America's leading cardiologists—is typical of the advice given to heart patients by orthodox medicine so far as heart disease is concerned:

> Nitroglycerin tablets, amyl nitrite perles, alcohol, and certain other drugs seem to dilate or cause the small coronary branches to relax, making the small vessels larger. People who have angina pectoris from effort are frequently able to prevent their pain by placing a nitro-glycerin tablet under the tongue just before doing a task which they know from experience will result in pain. For example, if a man must walk up a hill from the trolley every night when he comes from work, and he knows that if he walks up the hill he will have to stop a time or two because of pain, he may put a nitroglycerin tablet under his tongue as he gets off the trolley and go up the hill without pain. However, a better idea would be for the individual to move to another site, where there is no hill, or to go home by another route. Many people's lives have been made more comfortable by such compromises. A drink or two of brandy or whisky each day may be helpful in causing the arteries to dilate and is certainly not forbidden if the patient would like it. Following a coronary thrombosis, drugs that produce dilation of the small blood channels are given to speed the healing process.

The foregoing advice speaks for itself. As emergency therapy it may serve its purpose, but such treatment with drugs and alcohol as a general rule, inevitably makes the heart condition worse. Treatment on the lines indicated by Dr W. H. Gordon—which is common practice—has never been known to give any substantial or permanent improvement to a bad heart condition.

Drugs and heart ailments
The overall effects of drugs may be definitely harmful for

the heart. They fail to take into account the natural law that
'action and reaction are opposite and equal'. That is to say,
the drug that gives artificial stimulation to a feeble heart today
will do it at the price of greater enfeeblement tomorrow. That
dangerous policy leads to greater quantities of drugs to get
the same stimulation, and enfeeblement to the point of death
the moment the drugs are left off.

Many medical scientists now agree (1) that no heart ailment
was ever permanently cured by drugs; (2) that cure can only
be effected by fundamental changes in the body's nutrition
in general and by vitamin E in particular. Sir William Osler,
one-time Regius Professor of Medicine at Oxford university,
was fond of quoting Voltaire's indictment of drugs and
druggers: 'We put drugs, of which we know little, into bodies
which we know less, to cure diseases, of which we know
nothing at all.'

If you are now on drugs, it is almost certain that by carrying
out the dietary suggestions in this book which complement
the actions of drugs, you may eventually be able to reduce
your intake of these drugs. However, this should never be
done without the knowledge and agreement of your
practitioner because he is the only one able to monitor your
condition and determine what progress has been made.

4

Dietary Approaches
to Prevention of
Heart Disease

All the studies carried out over the last fifty years have shown quite conclusively that the development of coronary heart disease is related to dietary fat intake. This can be a direct effect due to high-saturated fat in the diet in its own right but this in turn affects the blood cholesterol levels. The major dietary influence on blood plasma LDL and total cholesterol is the amount and type of fat. There are over twenty studies in 14 countries indicating that high LDL and total blood plasma cholesterol is one of the big three risk factors for coronary heart disease. The other two are tobacco smoking (particularly cigarettes) and high blood-pressure.

The basic cause of narrowing of the coronary (and other) arteries is the development of atherosclerosis, a lesion of the artery wall characterized by a massive deposition of fat and blood products. Atherosclerosis by itself causes narrowing of the arteries but its particular significance in coronary heart disease is that a thrombus or clot almost always occurs in an artery that has already been affected by atherosclerosis. Coronary thrombosis, the sudden blockage of a coronary artery by a thrombus, causes the heart attack which can be fatal.

The course of atherosclerosis
In spite of the extent of research carried out there is still no agreement on the way in which atherosclerotic lesions are

initiated and develop in the artery wall. What is established is that fats and cholesterol in particular occur in all atherosclerotic lesions. All of that arterial cholesterol is derived from the blood but what is important is that the damaging level of fat and cholesterol in the blood can be altered by changing the composition of dietary fat.

Consumption of a Western-style diet high in animal fat is frequently associated with a high level of cholesterol in the blood. Studies of many populations throughout the world have shown that the blood cholesterol level is closely correlated statistically with mortality from coronary heart disease. Those with elevated blood cholesterol level, common amongst middle-aged men, are more likely to have a heart attack than those with a normal level. The risk rises progressively with higher blood cholesterol concentrations. Whilst this does not prove that a high blood cholesterol causes coronary heart disease it does suggest that a high blood cholesterol is an indication of increased chances of suffering a heart attack.

That there probably is a direct cause-and-effect relationship however, is, suggested by the following facts:
(1) Severe atherosclerosis is the underlaying pathological process in nearly all cases of coronary heart disease.
(2) Accumulation of cholesterol is a prominent feature of the developing atherosclerotic lesion.
(3) This cholesterol is derived from the blood.
(4) The risk of developing coronary heart disease is statistically associated with blood cholesterol level.
(5) In those populations where the general blood cholesterol level is low, severe atherosclerosis and coronary heart disease are rare, except perhaps in extreme old age.
(6) There is a high rate of coronary heart disease in middle age when the population eats diets high in saturated fats and cholesterol.

How do fats differ?

As a general rule, fats are hard and are derived from dairy products, animals and poultry. They are also produced artificially by chemically 'hardening' vegetable oils to produce hard margarines and cooking fats. The fatty acids that make up hard fats are saturated and those found mainly in our diets are lauric, myristic, palmitic and stearic. In addition to supplying saturated fatty acids, dairy products and meats from animals and poultry also provide cholesterol.

Vegetable oils are in the main composed of polyunsaturated fatty acids in which each carbon chain is deficient in four or more atoms of hydrogen so that two or more 'double bonds' are formed. The major sources of polyunsaturated fatty acids are corn (maize) oil, soyabean oil, sunflower seed oil and wheatgerm oil. We get these not only in liquid form but in their natural state as part of wholegrains and seeds that feature in some of our foods (unrefined cereals and mueslis). Amongst the common oils eaten, olive oil is the exception as its main constituent is oleic acid which is neither saturated nor polyunsaturated. Despite this, olive oil is eaten in vast quantities where coronary heart disease is no problem so it must have some protective factor in it even though we don't know what it is.

The most common polyunsaturated fatty acid in vegetable oils is linoleic acid and this is often referred to as an essential fatty acid. This is because its deficiency can lead to symptoms in animals that include skin disorders, failure to reproduce and eventually death. Now we know that these fatty acids are essential because the body cannot make them and they are precursors of body hormones called prostaglandins. We shall see later how these may be related to the development and prevention of coronary heart disease.

What is important, however, is that it has been known for at least twenty years that blood cholesterol levels can be reduced by substituting polyunsaturated fat (or oil) for saturated fats in the diet. It has been demonstrated many times that such a change in the diet is safe, practical and acceptable. The extent of the reduction in blood cholesterol level is related to the ratio of polyunsaturated to saturated fatty acids in the diet rather more than it does with the reduction of cholesterol intake. Of course, any reduction in animal fats in the food will not only decrease the saturated fat intake but also that of cholesterol. Hence the first priority in reducing blood cholesterol (and thus one's chances of suffering from coronary heart disease) is to reduce the saturated fats in the meals. Replacement of animal fats with polyunsaturated oils for cooking and for spreading (as polyunsaturated margarines) is also desirable.

General guidelines for reducing saturated fat and cholesterol in the diet with partial replacement by polyunsaturated fat are:

(1) Avoid butter and hydrogenated (hard) margarine, lard and suet. Use moderate amounts of polyunsaturated margarines.

(2) Avoid cream and ice-cream. Use skim or semi-skim (2 per cent fat) milk instead of standard, full cream milk.

(3) Eat less meat but more poultry and fish. Avoid the skin of poultry which is the main source of fat. Choose lean meat and remove visible fat. Grill rather than fry. Avoid sausages and meat pies.

(4) Reduce intakes of egg yolks. All cholesterol is in the yolk with none in egg white.

(5) Keep lard and cream cheese intakes down and use cottage cheese instead.

(6) Restrict your intake of cakes, pastries and biscuits (unless these are made with polyunsaturated oils and fats) and chocolates which are high in saturated fats.

(7) Use polyunsaturated oils for cooking, e.g. maize or sunflower oils. Ensure the brand you buy contains vitamin E.

(8) Eat more vegetables and fruits of all kinds. These foodstuffs are very low in every type of fat and supply high intakes of fibre at the same time. The only fats in vegetables are those that you add.

(9) Increase your intakes of cereals, bread, rice, pasta, breakfast cereals and oatmeal. Ensure they are the wholemeal variety or are unrefined. High complex polysaccharide (starch) foods like tapioca, cornflour and sago should also feature in your diet.

It is important to state yet again that the major dietary influence on plasma LDL cholesterol and total cholesterol is the amount and type of fat. The increased cholesterol effect comes mainly from the saturated fatty acids known as palmitic and myristic. Most diets contain more palmitic. Polyunsaturated fats, chiefly linoleic, tend to lower plasma LDL and total cholesterol but their effect is only half as strong as the elevating effect of palmitic acid. Hence any increase in polyunsaturated oil intake in the diet should be accompanied by a concomitant decrease in that of saturated fats—perhaps even complete replacement when possible. These effects on the cholesterol levels take between ten and fourteen days to appear and will last for as long as saturated fats are replaced by the polyunsaturated variety.

Dietary cholesterol: Other dietary constituents have a smaller effect. Eating cholesterol-rich foods like shellfish, liver, kidney and eggs in general has less effect on plasma cholesterol values than eating saturated fats. An egg contains about 250mg cholesterol so in most people there is little effect on plasma cholesterol, raising it by a mg or two only in 100cc of blood plasma. In about 20 per cent of the population though, there may be a greater rise so these are wise to abstain from cholesterol-rich foods altogether. There is regrettably no easy way of deciding who is in the 20 per cent responders apart from constant monitoring of blood plasma levels.

Reduced calorie intake: Loss of weight by reducing calorie intake can lower blood plasma cholesterol levels but it is more likely in those individuals who show both increased cholesterol and fat levels in their blood. There is no guarantee that such lowering will happen though. In anorexia nervosa where calorie intake approaches zero, the blood plasma cholesterol concentration is often raised.

Increased dietary fibre: The effect of increased dietary fibre on blood plasma cholesterol depends upon the type of fibre eaten. Insoluble fibres like bran have little or no effect upon the cholesterol level. Soluble fibres like guar gum, xanthan gum and pectin will cause major reductions in blood cholesterol levels but large amounts must be eaten. At a daily intake of 5g of a soluble fibre, cholesterol reduction can be as high as 5 per cent. As vegetables and fruits contain about 1 per cent pectin, four portions would provide about 5g soluble fibre. At the same time, increased intakes of high-fibre foods are likely to replace foods that are high in fat.

As a general dietary guideline, eat four servings of vegetables and fruit daily. One serving should be of the dark green, yellow or orange type such as leafy greens, broccoli, carrots, pumpkin, apricots, melon or mangoes. One serving should be from tomatoes or citrus or berry fruits. The other two servings should be of any other type of fruit or vegetables.

High-density lipoprotein cholesterol: This is the protective factor as it helps mobilize cholesterol from the tissues. Where there is a high incidence of coronary heart disease those with above average levels of HDL cholesterol have a reduced risk of developing the complaint. However, dietary fats have only a small effect on HDL. As we shall see later, vitamin supplementation can increase HDL cholesterol ratios in the blood. There are, however, greater proportions of HDL cholesterol in women than in men but those who are obese have the less desirable low proportion of this protective type of cholesterol. These observations could in part explain the reduced chances of heart attack in females and in the underweight.

The following countries all have expert committees who have recommended reductions in plasma cholesterol as a important factor in decreasing the chances of coronary heart disease: Australia, Canada, France, Holland, New Zealand, Scandinavia, UK, USA and West Germany.

Thrombosis: Diets that reduce the tendency to thrombosis are similar in many ways to those that lower blood plasma cholesterol, i.e. low in saturated fat. Such diets are of particular importance in preventing recurrence of a heart attack. In the young adult coronary heart disease is best prevented by the diets discussed above which lower plasma LDL cholesterol. In the older individual who may or may not have coronary heart disease similar dietary approaches may also be useful but in addition they should eat diets that make thrombosis less likely. Present knowledge suggests that fatty fish can do this.

A good indication of a person's chances of getting a thrombosis is the stickiness of their platelets, the small white blood cells that adhere together to form a blood clot. Any agent that reduces stickiness is therefore beneficial and the most potent inhibitors of thrombosis found in the diet are the fatty acids found in relatively high concentrations in fatty fish. Such conclusions are based on laboratory experiments and on observations on people, e.g. Eskimos, who subsist largely on fish.

Vegetable seed oils also have a similar inhibitory effect,

particularly those oils with high levels of linoleic acid, but the benefit is less pronounced than that with fish oils. It is also probable that the oils of garlic and onions contain some substance that reduces the process of thrombus formation so when these form a substantial part of the diet, as they do in some countries, the incidence of thrombosis is reduced. On the other hand, high-fat meals, high blood fats and high blood plasma cholesterol levels all favour thrombosis.

The heart muscle: This is known as the myocardium and it is susceptible to damage like any other muscle. However, it does appear to be especially sensitive to potassium deficiency both in the blood plasma itself and within the muscle cell walls. Lack of potassium makes the myocardium more easily damaged, prone to uneven heartbeats and more sensitive to digitalis. It is likely that sudden death after exercise is due to a sudden lowering of blood plasma potassium but why this should happen is not clear. What is apparent is that to maintain healthy potassium levels in the body we should ensure a good daily intake of fresh fruit, vegetables and their juices since these foodstuffs represent our best dietary sources of potassium. The dried varieties are even richer.

The effect of low magnesium levels may be mediated either through a lack of magnesium or an accompanying lack of potassium since both minerals tend to occur together in the same foods. Low magnesium in the myocardium is known to give rise to fast heartbeats that can also be irregular. In addition some people who had suffered heart attacks were also found to have low blood plasma magnesium levels. Hence any diet that contains both potassium and magnesium in any quantity is bound to have a beneficial effect upon heart muscle function.

Drinking water: The incidence of heart disease has been found to be lower in districts where the drinking water is hard than in those where it is soft. No one is sure what the protective factor in hard water is but various studies have indicated that magnesium or calcium is the most likely candidate. No matter what it is, a sensible precaution for anyone who has or is contemplating a water-softening system is to ensure that it is used only for their heating systems and tank water. Drinking water is best left hard if its beneficial effects on heart disease are to be retained.

A success story
A prime example of how controlling the above-mentioned factors can lead to a decrease in the incidence of coronary heart disease comes from North Karelia in Finland. This area is the most easterly county of Finland and in 1971 its population had the doubtful distinction of suffering the highest death rate from coronary heart disease in the world.

A community programme was therefore set up in which everyone was advised to stop smoking; eat less animal fats; eat more fruit and vegetables; avoid putting on weight and have their blood-pressure checked regularly. After eight years of these dietary and lifestyle measures, death from coronary heart disease had fallen by 24 per cent in men and by 51 per cent in women. These reductions were significantly greater than the general decline in coronary deaths in Finland as a whole during the same period. Here at last is positive proof that the dietary and other principles accepted by health-conscious people as contributing to healthy hearts, do so.

High blood-pressure and diet
High blood-pressure can be caused by many factors but in turn it is an important factor in determining the chances of getting coronary heart disease and a heart attack. It is

common not only in urban and industrialized people but prevalent in quiet Hebridean islands, in tropical Africa and in South Sea islands whose inhabitants cook in sea water. Let us now look at the dietary factors that are likely to give rise to high blood-pressure.

Salt: Although we may regard salt (sodium chloride) as the prime villain in increasing blood-pressure in some sectors of the population it is the sodium part of it that is believed to cause the damage. Sodium can of course be supplied from other sources (baking powder, monosodium glutamate, many drugs, food additives, food preservatives) but common salt is the way most of us get our main intake.

The evidence that salt intake correlates with the development of high blood-pressure is not difficult to find:

(1) In those countries whose populations have low salt levels in their diets (2g salt per day or less) high blood-pressure is not seen. On the other hand in Northern Japan, where salt intakes average 25g daily, there is the highest incidence of high blood-pressure and strokes in the world.

(2) Many individuals show a fall in blood-pressure when their salt intake is reduced. Diuretic drugs, which function by increasing sodium excretion, reduce the blood-pressure. Even without these drugs, reduced salt intake by not adding it at table, by omitting foods in which salt has been added during processing and by replacing such foods with low-salt varieties, can cause significant lowering of blood-pressure.

(3) In human experiments, increases in salt intakes have been found to cause small rises in blood-pressure.

How much salt? There is little doubt that most people eat salt not because they need it but for its effect on taste. In addition salt is still an important preservative for foods so such foods represent a rich source of sodium. As far as most people are concerned, the sodium naturally present in foods at levels of between 1 and 2g daily is sufficient for their needs. Only those who lose significant quantities of salt in their sweat because of heavy work or high temperatures may need more. Body needs are unlikely to be more than 1g per day.

For the general adult population, the USA and Australia and the WHO Expert Committee on Prevention of Coronary Heart Disease (1981) recommend that people should not eat more than 6g of salt per day. This supplies 2.3g of sodium.

As a general guide, high-sodium foods are ham, bacon, tongue, corned beef, salami, sausage, smoked fish, most refined breakfast cereals, baking powder, pickles, sauces, vegetable juices, soy sauce, anchovy paste, biscuits, cheese (especially blue-vein varieties), yeast and beef extracts, olives, canned vegetables, soups, pizzas, potato crisps. Foods that contain only medium levels of sodium are bread, cakes, milk, butter, margarine, low-salt cheeses, some mineral waters. Low-sodium foods include rice, oatmeal, plain wheatflour, pasta, coffee, tea, human milk, fruits (fresh, canned and dried), herbs, spices, alcoholic drinks, pepper, vinegar, cream, raw bran, and salt-free bread, butter, margarine and breakfast cereals. Evian, Perrier and Vittel mineral waters are virtually sodium-free.

Body weight: Obese people are likely to have higher blood-pressure than lean people. Normal weight people who do not eat enough food will lose weight and this is usually accompanied by a fall in their blood-pressure, even if it is normal. Typical blood-pressure reductions of 10mm systolic and 5mm diastolic pressure are seen for every 5kg (11lb) loss in weight in those who are both obese and hypertensive. This occurs even when sodium intake is not reduced.

Alcohol drinking: Heavy drinkers have higher blood-pressure than light drinkers or abstainers. This effect starts to be consistent above 4 drinks per day and increases steadily up to 8 drinks daily. Systolic pressure tends to be more affected than diastolic. One study on hospitalized alcoholics indicated an average fall of 20mm of systolic blood-pressure when these patients abstained from alcohol. Once drinking was resumed, the blood-pressure rose again.

Other food components that may lower blood-pressure

Vegetarian diets: One study carried out in Perth, Australia was on normal, healthy hospital staff members who were provided with all their meals as mixed animal/vegetable or vegetable only foods. Sodium intakes were kept the same. After six weeks each group of subjects was switched to the other diet. Blood-pressures were found to be significantly lowered by between 3.5 and 6.0mm by all subjects whilst they were on the vegetarian diet. The reasons were not clear but could have been related to the high potassium and magnesium levels in vegetarian diets and of course to the low-saturated fats in such diets.

Potassium: Vegetable foods contain more potassium than those derived from animal, fish and poultry sources. When potassium intakes in the diet are high, they can offset to some extent the blood-pressure increasing effect of sodium. High potassium foods include potatoes, pulses, instant coffee, dried fruits, treacle, fresh meat and fish, bran cereals, tomatoes, fresh fruit, beer, cow's milk, oatmeal, fruit juices, nuts, wines and vegetables. Low potassium foods include rice, chocolate, human milk, eggs, biscuits, bread, cheese, flour and refined cereals. Foods virtually devoid of potassium are sugar, jam, honey, butter, margarine, cream, vegetable oils and spirits.

A combination of high potassium-containing foods with the low-sodium varieties in the diet can make a positive contribution to reducing high blood-pressure or maintaining a normal one.

Magnesium: Increased intakes of magnesium can sometimes lower blood-pressure in hypertensive people. It is particularly effective when magnesium body levels have been depleted by drugs like diuretics. These drugs have the unfortunate side-effects of causing potassium and magnesium loss which can lower their effectiveness in reducing blood-pressure. Replacing both minerals allows the maximum blood-pressure-lowering effect to be maintained. Magnesium is distributed in foods in a somewhat similar manner to potassium. The richest sources are bran, wholegrain cereals, peas and beans. Refining and processing of all of these give rise to wholesale losses of magnesium, none of which are replaced by manufacturers. Hence high and prolonged intakes of such foods can be a contributory factor in the development of high blood-pressure.

Vegetable oils: The high polyunsaturated fatty acid oils like maize, sunflower, wheatgerm and soya can reduce high blood-pressure. When healthy people were changed from a diet predominant in saturated fats (contributing 40 per cent of the calories) to one with polyunsaturated oils (contributing only 23 per cent of the calories) their blood-pressure fell by 8mm systolic and 5mm diastolic. Another study on hypertensive people indicated even greater reductions in blood-pressure when polyunsaturated oils replaced animal fats in the diet.

The official view

In 1984, the Committee on Medical Aspects of Food Policy of the UK Department of Health and Social Security published a report by an expert panel on Diet and Cardiovascular Disease. The recommendations of the panel were concerned mainly with dietary changes to decrease the incidence of coronary heart disease and of sudden cardiac death. At the same time they pointed out that high blood-pressure is the main factor in cerebral thrombosis and stroke. The risk of high blood-pressure is increased by obesity, by high alcohol intake and by high-salt levels in the diet. Their recommendations are as follows:

(1) The consumption of saturated fatty acids (i.e. hard animal fats) and of fat in general should be decreased. They should supply no more than 15 per cent of the total food energy (1g of fat supplies 9 calories) with a total intake of fat of no more than 35 per cent of daily calories. At present, most Western diets supply between 40 and 45 per cent of the daily calories as fat. Vegetable oils, providing polyunsaturated fatty acids, should be sufficient to supply about 20 per cent of our daily calories. Remember that vegetable oils also provide 9 calories per gram. These recommendations do not apply to children of five and under.

(2) There are no recommendations about the dietary intake of cholesterol but if saturated animal fats are decreased, this will be accompanied by a parallel decrease in cholesterol intake.

(3) The consumption of simple sugars like sucrose (cane and beet sugar), glucose and fructose should not be increased further. We would go further and suggest keeping such sugars to a minimum in the diet since not only do they supply empty calories and lead to obesity but they lead to dental problems.

(4) Avoid excessive intakes of alcohol. This is defined as more than 100cc per day. Beer supplies up to 5 per cent alcohol; wines 9 to 13 per cent and spirits about 40 per cent alcohol.

(5) Dietary intake of common salt should not be increased further and steps should be taken to decrease it. Approximately 30 per cent of our salt intake is added during cooking and at the table. This can be decreased immediately. The other 70 per cent comes from food, much of it added during manufacture. Hence food manufacturers will have to change their methods but we can help ourselves by avoiding highly salted foods (look on the label).

(6) The intake of fibre-rich foods such as bread, cereals, fruit and vegetables should be increased. Remember that unrefined cereals, wholegrains and wholemeal flour are superior as providers of fibre to their refined forms.

(7) Obesity should be avoided by a combination of controlled food intake and regular exercise. Weight should be kept within the ranges specified in many official tables.

(8) The panel recommends that people should not smoke cigarettes.

Whilst these official recommendations are commendable, it is regretted that there are no positive suggestions about the consumption of vitamins and minerals. They do believe, however, that further studies are needed in respect of intake of vitamin D, selenium and magnesium in relation to heart diseases. In addition the World Health Organization suggests further studies on the possible role of minerals (particularly iodine and fluoride) in relation to heart complaints. Let us now look at how some studies have indicated an important role for vitamins and minerals and other essential constituents of the diet in reducing the possible development of heart and blood circulation problems.

5

Supplements for Heart Complaints

The fundamental cause of heart disease

Why have heart ailments increased so alarmingly in the last 100 years when most other diseases have been greatly reduced in incidence? This question was not answered really until 1948, when the Shute Foundation for Medical Research in Canada provided the explanation. The answer to the problem, briefly, is this: The basic cause of the alarming increase of heart disease is due to the refining of flour, a practice which began about ninety years ago and has increased with the years. When flour is refined two vital elements are removed—vitamin E and B complex vitamins. These vitamins are only to be found in the germ cell and the husk of the grain, respectively. The reason why flour is 'refined' was due to the discovery that the germ cell of wheat contains an oil which sent flour rancid after it had been stored for about three or four months. Remove the germ cells from the wheat with the husk and the flour would keep indefinitely. Thus treated, white flour could be sent to the ends of the earth without the danger of rancidity. The refining of flour, therefore, became the universal commercial practice. It seemed the logical and most economical way of handling and storing flour, the most basic food in the diet of man. But in their ignorance of vitamins, the millers dealt the health of civilized nations a mortal blow. The researches of the Shute Foundation have proved beyond doubt that:

(1) In removing the germ cell from wheat they also removed the richest known source of vitamin E, the muscle vitamin, which is essential for the maintenance of the vital heart muscle.

(2) In removing the husk from wheat they also removed the B group of vitamins—some twelve of them, which are essential to the nerve health of human beings.

And so it is that the white flour tradition has for nearly 100 years slowly, systematically and increasingly starved the people of their main source of vitamin E and the B group of vitamins. And so it is that, as a result of that long and systematic starvation, the most universal diseases today are (a) the breakdown of the powerful heart muscle and the subsequent crop of heart diseases—with one person in three dying of it. (b) The appalling crop of nervous disorders which have characterized the last half century as the most neurotic era in the world's history. Nearly half of all hospital cases today are mental cases. Every other bed in USA hospitals is now occupied by a mental patient.

Vitamin E

Dr Evan Shute on vitamin E

Dr Evan Shute, the principal of the Shute Foundation for Medical Research, enlarging on the way vitamin E works, has said:

> These functions of vitamin E, all of them extensively confirmed in animal experimentation and human clinical work, make it the most valuable ally the cardiologist has yet found in the treatment of heart disease. It has no rivals. No other substance has this array of needful properties. Vitamin E then becomes the first safe factor which can be given to patients suffering from the results of a clot in a coronary artery. There has been and still is no treatment at all for this type

of case, except two mildly useful drugs, which can be administered with great peril to the already precarious patient. Vitamin E replaces 'rest and reassurance', which have no authentic basis, with real help to the damaged, laboring heart itself. It is the key both to the prevention and treatment of all those conditions in which a lack of blood supply due to thickened or blocked blood vessels or a lack of oxygen is a major factor of the whole story of the disease. As I have said, it has no rivals. No pharmacologist or cardiologist can suggest another substance with all the powers and properties of this vitamin. God made it unique and we ignore it at our peril.

Work declared world famous:

This work is world famous. Some 96 medical papers, not including our own, have already been written in its support. How many does one need to win his case? Our work seems to have been the source of Ochsner's studies on the prevention of post-operative clotting by the use of vitamin E, of the work of many Italian workers on heart disease, of Professor Boyd's (of the University of Manchester) published treatment of intermittent claudication (Buerger's disease) and with phlebitis.

Over 160 medical men patients in institute:

We have over 160 medical men as personal patients at our institute. We know of many more who are taking it on their own. Presumably what is good enough for them is good enough for their patients. Early this month one appeared who had been a successful surgeon in California. After a heart attack he had been given vitamin E by his doctor. He merely came to us for regulation of his dosage. He used these words to me: 'Everybody is using it for the treatment of heart disease in California!'—A pleasant but slight exaggeration, perhaps. There is much animal experimentation to show that vitamin E may be the key to the control of hardening of the arteries.

I cannot help but recall the words of the great pathologist, Gideon Wells, under whom I studied pathology for 15 months, who told me that the man who discovered the prevention and treatment of arteriosclerosis had found the key to eternal youth. A man is as old or as young as his arteries. I would, if I had time, give you in detail the results of some of these experiments. I would like to tell you about the workers who showed that the deposits of cholesterol in the wall of the arteries in rabbits force-fed with cholesterol could be prevented by vitamin E.

Over 40,000 patients treated:

We have now personally treated over 40,000 cardiovascular patients. My great regret is that circumstances today prevent me from showing you some of our hundreds of coloured photographs of these people. I wonder how many people realize that this is many times the number seen in a comparable time elsewhere. We are no longer reporting on our first ten cases. We are reporting to you on the conclusions derived from thousands. It is an investigation that Canadians and Canada should be proud of, for in this at least they lead the world.

What vitamin E can improve it can also prevent! The truth is of the greatest importance to those many thousands of people who have not yet suffered a heart attack but who have had warnings that their hearts are heading for trouble. These people should begin taking vitamin E at once. Their dosage need only be two-thirds of the dosage required by angina cases namely 200mg daily but sufficiently high to help PREVENT such a deadly thing as a coronary occlusion—which is often fatal—happening to them. And for those people who are still in possession of sound hearts, with no symptoms whatever of heart trouble, it is a wise precaution for everybody past the 30 years mark to begin supplying the body with the vitamin E which they do not get in their daily food supply. They should begin the practice of taking 100mg per day which is low-cost insurance against heart disease in any of its lethal or crippling forms. From 40 to 60 years, 150mg daily is advisable, and after 60 years 200mg daily.

How vitamin E works

How does vitamin E bring about this amazing change for the better? It does so in a number of ways:

(1) Primarily, vitamin E is the 'muscle vitamin'. It dilates the capillary blood vessels, enabling the blood to flow more freely into muscle tissue, thus strengthening the muscle tissue and carrying blood more freely to the network of nerves throughout it.

(2) The significance of this will be more apparent when it is remembered that the heart is primarily a piece of muscle tissue—and the most important muscle in the body. Vitamin E—or rather, the alpha tocopherol in it—revitalizes and strengthens heart muscle that has deteriorated and restores it to more normal function. Its lesions are healed, and the heart is 'made over'.

(3) But vitamin E does much more than that. It decreases the oxygen requirement of muscle by over 40 per cent. Thus pain and breathlessness disappear and the sufferer is no longer exhausted by the slightest exertion. As Professors Houchin and Mattill have pointed out:

> This oxygen conserving mechanism in coronary heart disease is obviously of the greatest importance and probably explains the complete disappearance of angina pectoris in most patients on an adequate dosage of alpha tocopherol. It is really equivalent, as far as oxygenation is concerned, to increasing the blood supply to the heart—which is, of course, the fundamental corrective needed for proper cardiac function.

(4) Vitamin E also possess an anti-thrombin quality. That is to say, it prevents the clotting of blood in arteries and veins. But it does more, it dissolves blood clots. These qualities reduce the incidence of thrombosis.

(5) To quote Dr Evan Shute: 'It acts somehow upon both old fibrous heart tissue, as shown by Steinberg, of Rochester, and Burgess & Pritchard, of Montreal, and also upon the formation of new scar tissue.'

(6) It improves the whole circulatory mechanisms of the body in general and the heart in particular. 'Vitamin E' (alpha tocopherol), to quote Professors Hickman and Harris, 'is the most versatile and active of all the vitamins.' It is not surprising, therefore, that drastic changes for the worse develop in so many millions of human beings who are systematically starved of it. And it is equally not surprising that amazing changes for the better take place once vitamin E is systematically taken into the body.

The Vitamin E dosage

The dosage recommended by the Shute Foundation for Medical Research—which has made the effects of vitamin E on the heart its special study over several years—is as follows:

Coronary heart disease, including coronary occlusion and thrombosis:
Where the blood-pressure is not higher than 160 systolic, the dosage for this type of heart condition is 300 to 500mg of vitamin E daily, otherwise 200mg daily for the first four weeks. A routine practice is that one B complex tablet is taken with vitamin E during or immediately before each meal. To avoid danger of relapse, 300mg of vitamin E should be continued indefinitely, even after all heart symptoms have

disappeared. If after five weeks the heart symptoms have not disappeared, 500mg of vitamin E daily should be taken, or increased if necessary. The Shute Foundation stresses the importance of treating all cases of coronary occlusion (or thrombosis) immediately with 500mg of vitamin E. Owing to the unfortunate fact that most physicians are not yet acquainted with vitamin E therapy for cardiological cases, months, sometimes years, elapse before the patient starts on vitamin E. Had he commenced to take it immediately, his chances of recovery to better heart function would have been greatly increased.

Angina Pectoris: Where the blood-pressure is not higher than 160 systolic, the daily dosage should be 300 to 500mg of vitamin E. If higher, start on 100mg daily for four weeks, then increase by 50mg daily after each four weeks until 300mg or more daily are being taken.

Hypertrophy, endocarditis, myocarditis, pericarditis, mitral stenosis: These are heart conditions which respond to 300mg of vitamin E daily, plus one vitamin A capsule, one vitamin C tablet, 250mg, one B complex tablet, one B1 tablet (10mg) and one lecithin capsule, before each meal. Hypertensive heart disease—that is, heart symptoms complicated by high blood-pressure: 100mg vitamin E daily for one month; 120mg vitamin E daily for the second month; 150mg vitamin E daily for the third month; then the dosage should be lessened, maintained, or slowly increased by 20mg daily per month, according to the doctor's report. To quote the Shute Foundation:

> Of necessity the treatment of these cases is gradual and prolonged, but the results are very often satisfactory from the patient's standpoint. Indeed, relief of symptoms may be marked after the patient has been on 150 to 180mg of alpha

tocopherol (vitamin E) per day for a month or so, rarely on smaller dosage, and we often do not proceed to larger doses.

Diet for hypertension cases should be relatively salt-free on the lines set out in the dietetic section of the Science of Life booket, *High Blood-Pressure*. One B complex tablet is now routine practice, with the vitamin E dosage, before each meal, in every form of heart disorder. Lecithin capsules are also recommended (see later).

Acute rheumatic fever—the first attack:

If such cases are treated immediately with 400mg of vitamin E daily, irrespective of age, all evidence of disease may disappear in as little as three to seven days—at least by three to four weeks. Fever, joint symptoms and signs, tachycardia (excessive rapidity of the heart's action) will, in many a case, disappear entirely. We have had very few failures on such a schedule.

Drs W. E. and E. V. Shute,
on Alpha tocopherol in Cardiovascular Disease.

Continuing rheumatic fever with marked damage to the heart, with or without congestive failure, and with or without auricular fibrillation:

Here is a group in which we have rarely failed to obtain definite improvement, sometimes very striking and maintained for months, in each case with reduction of heart size, usually with disappearance or better control of the congestive failure, and with apparent inactivation of the disease. However, the damage is often enormous and all such patients face constant danger from intercurrent infections or sudden cardiac failure.

Shute Foundation.

Subsequent attacks of acute rheumatic fever in a latent case:

Herein the ideal treatment is 400mg vitamin E daily. There are some cases in which the damage from earlier attacks is so great that the full dosage cannot be given immediately. If heart size is nearly normal and heart damage moderate or relatively slight, we try full dosage. If damage is great we give 100mg daily for two weeks and then cautiously try full dosage. In a few cases we must treat these patients cautiously, giving 90mg per day for the first four weeks, 120mg daily for the second four weeks, and 150mg for the third four weeks, with increasing dosage if or as directed.

Shute Foundation.

Cautions

In serious heart ailments, the maintenance dosage equals the therapeutic dosage, and any reduction of the vitamin E dosage can result in a serious relapse. It cannot be too strongly emphasized that only the dosage indicated gets results. Attempts to get a moderate improvement with a moderate dosage invariably fail. The Shute brothers have warned that a half dosage is equal to NO DOSAGE. It is the alpha tocopherol content, according to the researches of the Shute Foundation for Medical Research, which plays the fundamental part in salvaging bad hearts and restoring them to normal function. Vitamin E is made up of alpha, gamma, beta, delta and three other tocopherols, but only alpha tocopherol has any therapeutical value. On this point the famous Shute Foundation for Medical Research, which has made Vitamin E its special research for several years, has written:

The only preparations of any value are those labelled in terms of alpha tocopherol since it is only the alpha tocopherol which has any therapeutic value. Therefore gamma, beta and delta tocopherols possess no value whatever in the treatment of cardio-vascular disease. They are inert members of the mixture of natural tocopherols which comprise vitamin E.

It is most important to use a reliable brand of vitamin E.

How safe is vitamin E?

When d-alpha tocopherol is administered orally in massive doses, it is well tolerated. No symptoms of toxicity have been reported in a number of species, including rats, mice, rabbits, dogs, cats and monkeys. An American study was published by the American Chemical Society in 1957. Adult volunteers were given levels as high as 500 to 600 i.u. vitamin E per kg body weight on a daily basis for five months with no recognizable symptoms of toxicity. This represents a daily intake of about 40,000 i.u. for an average 70 kg (11 st) adult.

There are, however, uncontrolled observations of possible untoward effects of large doses of vitamin E in small numbers of human subjects. In man the reported effects have always been minor and have never led to severe and permanent defects. If any side effects do occur, these can always be associated with the high vitamin E intake and cessation or reduction of the dose invariably removes the symptoms. For example one report in the *New England Journal of Medicine*(1973) mentions that a dose of 800 i.u. per day for one week induced a weakness and fatigue in one person, rather like the symptoms of influenza. Reducing the intake to 400 i.u. per day caused no ill-effect and this dose was easily tolerated for long periods.

Other reports in the *Journal of the American Medical Association* (1974) found no ill-effects in a number of patients treated with 800 i.u. of the vitamin per day. At much larger doses there was reversible muscle weakness, disturbed reproductive functions and gastro-intestinal upsets.

Typical symptoms of vitamin E excess are muscle weakness and proneness to fatigue. Other signs of over-dosage include rising blood-pressure and palpitations of the heart. Sometimes the high concentration of oil gives rise to mild diarrhoea and nausea but these are not noted with the water-solubilized forms. Biochemical changes may cause the raised creatine level in the urine mentioned before.

Like other fat-soluble vitamins, the symptoms of vitamin E excess are similar to those of its deficiency. However, these are simply warning signs and a reduction of dosage to a level where these symptoms are not produced indicates that amount of vitamin E which the body can tolerate.

An expert panel on Food Safety and Nutrition said in the publication Food Technology in 1977 'There is no evidence that the tocopherols are toxic, even in large doses.' A leading article in *The Lancet* in 1974 concluded that 'Vitamin E is a natural nutrient; administration leads to no toxic effects.'

In rare cases there may be an effect of vitamin E upon other medical treatments. There is one case on record of a man having anticoagulant therapy for blood clotting problems, whose vitamin K levels decreased during therapy with 1,200 i.u. of vitamin E per day. A low vitamin K concentration in the blood leads to an increase in the length of time it takes the blood to clot. Once the vitamin E was stopped, the concentration of vitamin K dependent coagulating factors returned to normal and a normal blood-clotting time was resumed. This effect indicates the anti-thrombotic (i.e. anti-blood clotting) property of vitamin E. Large doses of alpha tocopherol in anaemic children may suppress the normal blood-forming response to injected iron. This, however, represents no problem once the deficient factor causing the anaemia has been identified.

Thiamine (vitamin B1)

Thiamine is essential for a healthy heart. Dr J. B. Sutherland of the University of Ottawa School of Medicine found that lack of vitamin B1 in rats caused slowed heartbeats, enlarged hearts and eventual heart failure. These findings are related to a heavy dependence of the heart on the vitamin for its energy production. In man, studies reported in *Nutrition Reviews* (October 1955) revealed that the thiamine contents of heart muscle from those patients dying of heart failure were lower than those who had healthy diets but had died from other causes. The most likely cause was felt to be a prolonged inadequate intake of the vitamin in the patient's diet. This conclusion was also reached by Prof. E. Cheraskin writing in the *Journal of the American Geriatrics Society* (1967) who studied the problem from a different approach. He measured the intakes of thiamine in healthy human beings, then followed their medical history. Those with the lower intakes ended up with twice the number of heart problems of those taking the higher amounts in their food. An extension of this trial revealed that the lower intake of the vitamin B1 was associated with a higher intake of refined carbohydrate. This was felt to be the prime factor in the development of a mild deficiency of vitamin B1.

Thiamine is perfectly safe when given orally in amounts totalling hundreds of milligrams. Occasional toxicity has been reported, but only when the vitamin was given intramuscularly or intravenously by injection.

Nicotinic acid (vitamin B3)

Reducing the blood cholesterol
Nicotinic acid, but not nicotinamide, will reduce cholesterol levels in the blood. In a short-term trial at the Mayo Clinic in 1956, 3g of nicotinic acid were given orally to patients with high blood cholesterol and levels were lowered to normal in 72 per cent of those tested. The remaining 28 per cent responded favourably to 4-6g per day. A longer term study

over eleven years was carried out at the Dartmouth-Hitchcock Medical Centre in New Hampshire. A dose of 100mg nicotinic acid was given to 160 patients after each meal and this was increased over eleven days to 1g after each meal, at which level therapy continued. The average decrease in plasma cholesterol was 26 per cent in those who took the vitamin for at least one year, and the lower cholesterol level was maintained for as long as treatment continued. It was particularly gratifying to note that these were no serious side-effects.

Other studies in Britain have indicated that nicotinic acid also has the property of lowering blood fats (triglycerides) in general in the above doses. In this respect it appears to be as effective as the drug clofibrate. It is believed to act in two ways: first, by inhibiting the synthesis of fats in the blood; and second, by competing with and preventing the release of free fatty acids which combine with cholesterol.

Nicotinic acid causes blood vessels to dilate and so, when given in large doses, it may cause flushing of the face, a sensation of heat and a pounding headache. These symptoms are of a transient nature but can be distressing to some.

Other toxic symptoms reported with high doses of nicotinic acid include dry skin, rashes, itching and boils. Abdominal cramps, diarrhoea and nausea sometimes appear. An increase in blood uric acid leading to mild gout symptoms occasionally result from 6g of nicotinic acid taken on a regular basis. All these symptoms disappear when treatment with the vitamin ceases. Such high doses of nicotinic acid should not be taken by anyone suffering from gastric or duodenal ulcers since the vitamin in this form can irritate the ulcer. The record for excessive intake of nicotinic acid must belong to a patient of Dr A. Hoffer. He took 90g in a suicide attempt, but the only result was nausea, vomiting and diarrhoea.

Pyridoxine (vitamin B6)

An amino acid that depends upon vitamin B6 for its metabolism in the body is L-methionine. This material is converted to homocysteine which is a toxic compound. Under normal circumstances this does not matter because it, in turn, is converted very quickly into cystathionine, a very important amino acid needed for other body actions. The change from homocysteine to cystathionine is dependent upon vitamin B6. Some unfortunate individuals are born with a hereditary defect that means they are unable to make this change, with the result that they are mentally retarded and rarely live beyond their teens. However, it is very interesting that these young people have extensive disease of the blood vessels which are thickened by the deposition of fatty plaques—a condition known as atherosclerosis. It looks as though the build-up of excessive homocysteine prematurely gives rise to this disease which is usually reserved for middle and old age.

These findings led Dr Kilner McCully working at Harvard University and the Massachusetts General Hospital to suggest in 1969 that high concentrations of homocysteine induced by a deficiency of vitamin B6 may help to cause atherosclerosis. This conclusion was based not only on his own findings, but also on research carried out elsewhere. For example, Drs James Rinehart and Louis Greenberg of the University of California Medical School fed monkeys a diet deficient in vitamin B6. The animals developed atherosclerosis. No other B vitamin deficiency induced the condition. Other observations include: first, when human beings and animals develop vitamin B6 deficiency, the level of the toxic homocysteine in the blood rises; second, worldwide studies indicate that those suffering from atherosclerosis invariably have low vitamin B6 levels in their blood; and third, those people with atherosclerosis have high levels of homocysteine in their blood. There may also be a relationship between the B6 deficiency known to be induced by the 'Pill' and the increased occurrence of heart and blood vessel disease known to exist in those women taking this form of contraception. An English study of 46,000 women who had taken the 'Pill' for at least five years indicated that they had an incidence of heart and blood vessel disease some ten times greater than that associated with a similar number of women who practised other forms of contraception. The evidence is suggestive, but not conclusive, since their vitamin B6 status was not measured.

It is tempting, then, to suggest that atherosclerosis is another disease related to vitamin B6 deficiency, particularly when this may occur throughout a lifetime of bad dietary habits. Whilst the academics work out the mechanisms, however, it is perhaps safer simply to ensure against even a mild deficiency of vitamin B6 by eating the right foods and taking supplements where food alone cannot guarantee an adequate intake as in those taking the 'Pill'.

Recent reports suggest that vitamin B6 can be toxic in very high doses. However, in none of the clinical trials where doses did not exceed 200mg daily were toxic effects reported. Most people, however, are unlikely to need more than 25mg daily to help maintain healthy hearts. With other conditions such as Premenstrual Tension or for those taking the 'Pill', more may be needed but is unlikely to exceed 50mg daily. Some may prefer 100mg but if this dose does not help, neither is a more potent one. Under medical supervision, of course, higher intakes may be taken.

Choline, inositol and lecithin

Choline: an anti-fat agent

Choline is defined as a lipotropic factor which means that

it prevents fats from accumulating in the liver by facilitating the transport of those fats to the organs that require them. Liver normally contains only between 5 and 7 per cent of its weight as fat, but in the absence of choline this proportion can increase to as much as 50 per cent. Such fatty deposits, when allowed to build up in the vital organ, adversely affect its normal functioning and the ill-effects are soon felt. There are a number of diseases that can give rise to fatty liver and these include diabetes, alcoholism and protein-deficiency. Lack of choline has been implicated in the development of fatty liver by Dr S. Mookerjea of the University of Toronto, who observed an increase of liver fats during periods of choline deprivation.

When fats are transported from the liver, they do so in the form of complex substances called phospholipids. These are composed of fats, phosphorus, sugar and choline in combination. According to experimental evidence from animal work published in the *American Journal of Clinical Nutrition* (1965), lack of choline prevented this mechanism from operating with the result that the liver cells soon filled up with unwanted fat. Supplementation with choline not only prevented such changes but actually reversed the process and cleared the liver of accumulated fat. Human studies on infants suffering from fatty liver (*Journal of American Medical Association*, 1951) have confirmed a similar role for choline in human beings.

Control of blood-pressure

It is possible that prolonged low levels of choline in the body can give rise to high blood-pressure (hypertension). The compound was given to a group of patients suffering from hypertension with beneficial results according to a report in *Journal of Vitaminology* (1957). Typical symptoms of palpitations, dizziness and headaches disappeared within two weeks of treatment, together with reduction of the blood-pressure to normal. The mechanism of this action is not known, but it could be via the nerves controlling the blood vessels, which in turn determine the blood-pressure. Other evidence suggests that low levels of choline throughout life may put some individuals on the road to hypertension in later years.

Where do we obtain choline?

Choline is widely distributed in plants and animals and the richest sources include brewer's yeast, fish, soyabeans, nuts, liver, eggs and wheatgerm. Choline usually occurs as a component of phospholipids, complexes of fatty acids, phosphorus, sugar and choline. The most abundant phospholipid is lecithin and this represents one of the richest sources of choline.

There have been some measurements of choline in foods and these include: egg yolk, 1,700mg per 100g (there is none in egg-white); meat, 600mg per 100g; brewer's yeast, 300mg per 100g; and pure lecithin, which contains an average of 3,430mg per 100g. Daily intake from an average diet has been calculated as between 500mg and 1,000mg. The significance of the daily requirements is obscure since the body is probably capable of synthesizing its needs from other food materials. However, there are examples of complaints that have responded to extra choline in the diet which suggests that body synthesis may not always be sufficient.

Diseases of fat metabolism

The role of choline in ensuring mobility of fat and maintaining it in solution has lead to its use in diseases where fat metabolism has gone wrong. In the *Proceedings of the Society of Biology and Medicine* (1950), Drs L. M. Morrison and W. F. Gonzalez reported beneficial effects of choline treatment in patients suffering from atherosclerosis—a condition where the blood vessels become thickened by the deposition of fat. In the form of lecithin, choline has also been used successfully in those suffering from angina, thrombosis and stroke. Any condition that may be related to a high blood cholesterol and fat content is often helped by choline supplementation. It must be stressed, however, that choline is usually given in the form of lecithin in these cases. This is because lecithin also contains unsaturated fatty acids which contribute to the beneficial action of choline in any upset of fat metabolism.

Inositol: A fat-fighter

We have seen above how important choline is as a lipotropic agent in ensuring that fat is kept in solution and is not deposited in the wrong places in the body. The second factor that also has this property is inositol, but it is structurally very different from choline and hence exerts its lipotropic action in a different way. The fat-fighting properties of inositol appear to act in addition to those associated with choline, so it is not surprising that both are essential in controlling fat metabolism. There are reports from the American Heart Journal, 1949, by Drs I. Leinwand and D. H. Moore that given 3g of inositol daily to atherosclerotic patients resulted in a reduction of blood fats and cholesterol. Similar treatment reduced the excessive deposition of fat in those suffering from fatty liver. Despite these early reports, however, it is now accepted that the best way to restore fat metabolism to normal is by treating with both choline and inositol. Drs D. A. Sherber and M. M. Levites reported in the *Journal of the American Medical Association* in 1953 that this approach was successful in reducing cholesterol levels in all their patients subjected to the treatment.

Inositol is widely distributed in plants and animals with

the richest sources recognized as beef brain, beef heart, wheatgerm, wholegrains, brown rice, nuts, brewer's yeast and citrus fruits.

Lecithin

Lecithin supplies inositol as well as choline, and in a similar amount. In fact, it is highly likely that the anti-fat actions of choline and inositol reside in their presence in the lecithin molecule. With ample supplies of choline and inositol in the food, the body is capable of incorporating both of them into lecithin. Similarly, it can utilize both compounds when they are fed as lecithin. It is likely that, to obtain the maximum benefit, at least as far as their fat-fighting qualities are concerned, the lecithin should be from plant sources e.g. soya.

Daily intakes of inositol are probably similar to those of choline within the range 500 to 1,000mg. Therapeutic doses can go higher than this with no fear of side-effects. It is preferable to take inositol as plant lecithin because of the beneficial effects of the accompanying choline and unsaturated fatty acids.

Lecithin capsules taken regularly can help prevent the onset of heart diseases. For those suffering from such complaints or those with high blood-pressure, higher doses taken as the pure lecithin granules are preferred. One teaspoonful to one tablespoonful can be taken with each meal depending upon the severity of the condition.

Vitamin C

Reduces High Blood Cholesterol

When guinea-pigs are deprived of vitamin C, cholesterol levels increase in the blood, and fats are deposited in the walls of blood vessels, particularly those of the heart and brain. These animals also show a greater tendency to form gallstones.

Most gallstones in any species, including man, are composed of cholesterol and they tend to form by precipitation when bile cholesterol levels increase. This is precisely what happens in the C-deficient guinea-pigs. Modern research suggests that vitamin C has an important function in controlling blood cholesterol and fat levels in human beings also.

The leading researcher in this field is Dr E. Ginter of the Institute of Human Nutrition Research, Bratislava, Czechoslovakia. He studied the relationship between vitamin C levels in the white blood cells and the concentration of cholesterol and fats in the blood of a large number of patients, both male and female. The highly significant result to emerge, was that the lower the vitamin C level in these people, the higher were the cholesterol and blood fat levels. The next stage was to determine if cholesterol and fat levels could be reduced by increasing the vitamin C intake and this is exactly what Dr Ginter found. Diabetic patients (who usually have high blood cholesterol), and others who had high blood cholesterol levels with no obvious causes, were treated with 500mg vitamin C per day. The blood cholesterol levels and the total fat in the blood were reduced in all cases. This reduction was maintained while those patients were given ample vitamin C. Similar supplementation on a group of patients who did not have high cholesterol levels had no effect. In other words, ascorbic acid will reduce excessive cholesterol, but once normal levels are achieved it has no further influence.

How does vitamin C achieve cholesterol reduction? It increases the rate at which cholesterol is converted into bile acids and hence excreted. In his patients Dr Ginter found no evidence of a higher excretion of cholesterol as such, but what did increase dramatically was their excretion of bile acids. The usual route through which the body disposes of cholesterol is to convert it into bile acids in the liver, which are then deposited in the bile, carried to the intestine where they assist in fat digestion and end up excreted in the faeces. Speeding up this process neatly disposes of excess cholesterol. Drugs that decrease cholesterol usually do so by preventing its synthesis by the body. Recently, however, these drugs have received adverse publicity because of their serious side-effects. It looks now as though we have in vitamin C a safe, effective treatment that works in a more logical manner, by accelerating the disposal of cholesterol. Blood fats are also reduced by vitamin C, but although the mechanism is not completely worked out, the vitamin is just as effective and safe.

There may be other benefits from an intake of 500mg of ascorbic acid daily. Dr Geoffrey Taylor, formerly professor of medicine at the University of Lahore, has reported that changes in the tiny blood vessels, particularly those under the tongue, may be the warning signs of impending stroke. These changes also appear in scurvy and in mild deficiency of vitamin C. The number of deaths from strokes and coronary heart disease increase in cold weather in the winter, when the need for ascorbic acid is highest, but intake is at its lowest. Dr Constance Lesley of the Wakefield Group of Hospitals in Yorkshire is another expert who has found that vitamin C exerts a powerful protective effect on certain high-risk groups of the population. It could help prevent heart attacks, strokes, deep vein thrombosis and atherosclerosis through its fat-controlling function as described by Dr Ginter.

We know that fat is only one factor in increasing the risks of these conditions. Stress, diet, smoking and alcohol also may contribute. Yet we have seen that all of these may lower the vitamin C levels of the body by poor intake or excessive destruction or increased requirements of the vitamin. Vegetarians who have a high intake of vitamin C and various other groups who, for religious or ethical reasons, do not partake of the lifestyle dictated by the other factors, all have lower incidence of the diseases mentioned. Perhaps we should all look to our vitamin C intakes as one of the sensible means to reduce the chances of these blood-related diseases.

Fish body oils

The most exciting recent research development in the prevention and treatment of heart conditions is that concerning the use of fish body oils and in some cases fish liver oils. The fish that confer these benefits are the fatty variety including eel, herring, bloater, kipper, mackerel, pilchard, salmon, sardines, sprats, trout, tuna, whitebait and menhaden. White fish are less effective. Let us look first at the historical background to these studies.

Early evidence: The Eskimos share with the Japanese the advantage of a very low rate of death from coronary heart disease. Eskimos have diets very high in fats because of their high intakes of fatty fish and seal meat. Japanese too eat a lot of fish yet despite high levels of fats in their food both peoples do not appear to suffer the heart problems we associate in the West with rich fatty diets. The fundamental difference between the diets, however, is that most of the fat on which Eskimos and Japanese live is derived from fatty fish. Fish fats confer benefits not associated with animal fats.

The difference is seen in Japanese fishermen who consume 250g fish daily compared with only 90g per day in Japanese farmers. One distinction between the two groups was in the viscosity of their blood. Fishermen had lower viscosity (thin blood) than the farmers, whose blood was 'thick'. It is generally accepted that thinning of the blood reduces the chances of thrombosis.

Eskimo diets were even richer in fish intakes, reaching up to 500g per day as a staple diet. It is highly significant that once Eskimos leave their traditional way of life and eat a Western diet, their rate of coronary heart disease increases to that of those in the West. Japanese who emigrate to the USA show a similar inclination towards heart diseases in the West once they establish Western ways.

The protective factors of fish body oils

All fats and oils are composed mainly of fatty acids and we have seen that in terms of health, polyunsaturated fatty acids are the desirable type. The body oils of fatty fish are, however, rich in two particular polyunsaturated fatty acids that are not found in animal fats nor vegetable oils to any great extent. These are called eicosapentaenoic acid (EPA) and docosahexaenoic acid (DHA). Fish-eaters like the Japanese fishermen and Eskimos take in about 2.6g of EPA in their diets compared with only 0.9g in the farming community. These dietary differences were reflected in the blood fats of the fish eaters which were much higher in EPA and DHA levels. To see how these fatty acids do confer some protection against heart disease, let us look at some of the experimental work carried out on human beings.

Dr Von Lossonoczy and his colleagues reported in the *American Journal of Clinical Nutrition* (1978) that when they fed subjects a daily portion of 200g of mackerel (8g EPA) or of 150g cheese as well as other normal dietary fat intakes, the blood serum cholesterol fell from 216 to 197mg per 100ml; blood fats reduced from 80.4 to 55.2mg per 10ml and HDL cholesterol rose from 55.2 to 58.9mg to 100ml in those on the mackerel diet. When the subjects reverted to a cheese diet, all figures returned to the original undesirable ones.

Mackerel was also used in a study by Dr Liess and colleagues reported in *The Lancet* (1980). Volunteers were fed between 500 and 800g stewed or smoked mackerel daily for one week. The researchers found that there were marked changes in the capacity of the blood to form a thrombosis. This was much lessened on the fish diet.

A comprehensive study by Drs Harris and Connor (*Transactions of the Association of American Physicians*, 1980), who fed volunteers a diet high in salmon oil, reported that in their subjects there were significantly lower levels of blood cholesterol, VLDL cholesterol, LDL cholesterol and total blood fats. Although HDL cholesterol was not altered, the lowering in LDL cholesterol created a favourable HDL:LDL ratio. Whilst on the salmon diet, blood fats were cleared away from the blood much more quickly and the blood thinned considerably, reducing the chances of thrombosis significantly.

People who deliberately partake of an Eskimo diet (e.g. Prof. Hugh Sinclair of Oxford) for as little a period as six weeks noted profound differences in their blood fats and the ability of the blood to clot. In all cases VLDL cholesterol was reduced with a concomitant increase in HDL cholesterol. There was a pronounced 'thinning of the blood'.

Many other studies have shown beneficial results by feeding fatty fish, fish body oils or cod liver oil but all were healthy people. When those suffering from heart disease were studied the benefits were such to improve their lives. Dr A. M. Nelson, an American physician from Seattle, USA, has treated his heart patients with fish diets from 1972 and has claimed substantially longer survival times for these patients far beyond those expected (*Geriatrics*, December 1972).

Studies in the UK on fish body oils in heart patients have indicated a lowering of blood fats and cholesterol levels with a general improvement in the health of the patients, particularly those with angina (Cardiac Unit, Sheffield General Hospital). The diets of these people were controlled to reduce their intakes of animal fats and the fish oils were presented as MAXEPA capsules (up to ten per day), each capsule containing 1,000mg of oil with 180mg EPA and 120mg DHA.

How do fish body oils work?

No one is absolutely certain how the fatty acids in the fish body oils EPA and DHA confer their beneficial actions but a lot of evidence is now building up to such an extent that a reasonable hypothesis can be put forward. It has been established that both fatty acids are precursors of important hormones in the body called prostaglandins. Whilst there are dozens of prostaglandins being formed within the body daily, two of them concern us here as they function in the production of thrombi or blood clots.

One prostaglandin metabolite is called thromboxane and it is made within the tiny white blood cells called platelets. Thromboxane stimulates the formation of thrombi. Another prostglandin metabolite is called prostacyclin and it is produced continuously by the inside walls of blood vessels and their tissues. Prostacyclin has properties that inhibit thrombus formation and hence its role is to neutralize the effect of thromboxane.

The all-important condition for healthy blood is therefore a correct balance between thromboxane and prostacyclin with the desired ratio towards prostacyclin. The most important precursors of prostacyclin are EPA and DHA, so as long as these are provided from a fatty fish diet or from fish body oils the balance is towards high prostacyclin levels. Thromboxane is produced from other types of polyunsaturated fatty acids which also feature in the diet. All types of polyunsaturated fatty acids (and hence the prostaglandins produced from them) are essential because they have other important functions but it is necessary to maintain a balance amongst them. If thromboxane is allowed to dominate, the chances of thrombus formation are increased. With a bias towards prostacyclin, the chances of thrombus formation are decreased. Fatty fish diets (or capsules) hence keep our balance towards the desirable prostacyclin. Cod liver oil has similar beneficial properties but the amount required (a tablespoonful three times daily) is dangerous because of the high levels of vitamins A and D that such a volume supplies. However, cod liver oil without the vitamins but with the desirable EPA and DHA is now available.

This is still only a working hypothesis about how a fish diet can benefit us in our prevention and treatment of heart problems but it is becoming more and more likely as research proceeds. It may be over-simplified but whilst the researchers work out the mechanisms, there is a clear message to the rest of us. Incorporate fatty fish in your diet at least twice a week as a main course and supplement your diet with fish body oils or devitaminized cod liver oil daily. At the same time, the other dietary suggestions in this book should be adhered to.

The seven remedial principles
Once we understand the causes of a human ailment, we are half-way to curing it. By reversing the seven causes and by applying the curative principles consistently, 80 out of every 100 heart sufferers can not only rid themselves of distressing—indeed, alarming—heart symptoms, and the serious limitations that accompany them, but can gradually regain a high standard of health they may not have enjoyed for many years.

Here are the seven steps to achieve these objectives:

(1) Supply the heart muscle with vitamin E, the lack of which has been largely responsible for its deterioration and its disease.

(2) Take three B complex vitamin tablets daily to restore

nerve health in general and reduce the nervous tension of the heart in particular. One or two vitamin C (250mg) tablets should also be taken to build robust, healthy walls for the veins and arteries, enabling them to cope with the flow of blood without weakening. Vitamin C also helps to build strong connective tissue, and destroys bacteria that invade the blood-stream.

(3) Arrange one's diet so that it consists of vital foods. Cut out the 'foodless' foods which are listed below, and follow (as closely as possible) the ideal diet for heart cases.

(4) Reduce the protein, sugary, and fatty foods to the minimum. Most heart cases are the better for cutting out fat meat, eggs, and animal fats. But if you are not prepared to do that, reduce meat and eggs to one small serving each day. Substitute cheese as your main protein occasionally. It has a better protein value than meat or eggs and is rich in calcium, which is essential for the health of the bone structure and the nerves. Use fatty fish as your main protein twice a week.

(5) Eat less—much less. Most heart sufferers are overweight—a fact which puts an added strain upon the heart in pumping blood throughout a circulatory system entombed in fat.

(6) Gradually restore the body to better physical tone by moderate exercise and skin massage.

(7) Cut out cigarette smoking, which constricts the blood vessels.

Reject these pseudo foods

Here is a list of 'foodless' foods that no heart patient should eat. These are the 'foods' which create the fatty deposits that silt up the circulatory mechanism:

    White bread

    White-flour products, including pies and cake

Sugar—white or brown
Processed breakfast foods—flaked, 'puffed' or refined
Pastry and biscuits
Confectionery
Excessive servings of animal fats
Sausage meat
Corned meat, pickled and tinned meat
Fried foods
Re-heated and re-cooked soups, meat and vegetables
Pickled vegetables
Salt, and salty foods
Strong tea and coffee, soft drinks
Condiments of all descriptions
Jam
Most packeted and tinned foods, 'Instant' foods
All 'puddings', indeed all desserts other than fruit, stewed
    fruit, junket or yogurt.

The above 'foodless foods' cause most of the ills to which
the flesh is heir. They are responsible for saturating the tissues
with acid end-products and for silting up the vascular
(circulatory) system with uric acid deposits and cholesterol.
They may be the cause of glandular malfunction, which slows
up the whole governing mechanism of the body. In short,
the long-term effect of these alleged foods is homicidal. The
wise man and woman will wipe them off the dietetic list,
not only for the duration of the treatment, but for the duration
of life.

Index

(Entries in **bold** type refer to illustrations.)